Modification of Lipid Metabolism

Modification of Lipid Metabolism

Edited by

Edward G. Perkins
Department of Food Science
University of Illinois
Urbana, Illinois

Lloyd A. Witting
Denton, Texas

Academic Press, Inc.
New York San Francisco London 1975
A Subsidiary of Harcourt Brace Jovanovich, Publishers

ACADEMIC PRESS, INC.
111 Fifth Avenue, New York, New York 10003

United Kingdom Edition published by
ACADEMIC PRESS, INC. (LONDON) LTD.
24/28 Oval Road, London NW1

Library of Congress Cataloging in Publication Data

Main entry under title:

Modification of lipid metabolism.

"Symposium, held at the American Chemical Society
meeting in Atlantic City, New Jersey, September
10-11, 1974."
    Bibliography: p.
    Includes indexes.
    1.   Lipid metabolism—Congresses.   2.   Lipid
metabolism disorders—Congresses.   I.   Perkins,
Edward George,   (date)   II.   Witting, Lloyd Allen,
(date)   III.   American Chemical Society.
[DNLM: 1.   Lipid—Metabolism, Inborn errors—Congresses.   2.   Lipid—Metabolism.   QU85 A512m 1974]
QP751.M6   612'. 397   75-32542
ISBN 0—12—551150—7

PRINTED IN THE UNITED STATES OF AMERICA

Contents

CONTENTS

Inborn Errors of Lipid Metabolism and Lysosomal Storage Disorders

Michel Philippart

Intervention in Sphingolipid Metabolism with Synthetic Inhibitors

Norman S. Radin, Kenneth R. Warren, Ramesh C. Arora, Jung C. Hyun, and Radhey S. Misra

Modification of Membrane Glycolipids by Oncogenic Agents

Peter H. Fishman and Roscoe O. Brady

CONTENTS

Dietary Regulation of Lipid Metabolism

Dale R. Romsos and Gilbert A. Leveille

Effect of (–)-Hydroxycitrate on Lipid Metabolism

Ann C. Sullivan

Early Nutritional Influences on Development

M. R. C. Greenwood

The Influence of Environmental Factors on Lipid Metabolism

A. Saari Csallany and Roger I. Brooks

The Effect of Temperature Changes on Lipids and Proteins of Biological Membranes

Roland C. Aloia and George Rouser

List of Contributors

Numbers in parentheses indicate the pages on which the
authors' contributions begin.

Roland C. Aloia, (225) Department of Biology, University of California
Riverside, California

Ramesh C. Arora, (87) Department of Biochemistry, Chicago School of
Medicine, 2020 West Ogden Avenue, Chicago, Illinois

Joyce L. Beare-Rogers, (43) Bureau of Nutritional Sciences, Department of
Health and Welfare, Ottawa, Canada

Roscoe O. Brady, (105) Developmental and Metabolic Neurology Branch,
National Institute of Neurological Diseases and Stroke, The National
Institutes of Health, Bethesda, Maryland

Roger I. Brooks, (197) Department of Food Science and Nutrition, University
of Minnesota, St. Paul, Minnesota

A. Saari Csallany, (197) Department of Food Science and Nutrition, University
of Minnesota, St. Paul, Minnesota

Peter H. Fishman, (105) Developmental and Metabolic Neurology Branch,
National Institute of Neurological Diseases and Stroke, The National
Institutes of Health, Bethesda, Maryland

M. R. C. Greenwood, (175) Institute of Human Nutrition, College of Physicians
and Surgeons, Columbia University, New York, New York

Jung C. Hyun, (87) Neuroscience Laboratory Building, 1103 Huron, University
of Michigan, Ann Arbor, Michigan

Gilbert A. Leveille, (127) Department of Food Science and Human Nutrition,
Michigan State University, East Lansing, Michigan

Radhey S. Misra, (87) Michigan Cancer Foundation, Bio-organic Laboratories, 110 East Warren Avenue, Detroit, Michigan

Michel Philippart, (59) Mental Retardation Research Center, Department of Pediatrics, Psychiatry and Neurology, University of California- Los Angeles, Los Angeles, California

Norman S. Radin, (87) Mental Health Research Institute, University of Michigan, Ann Arbor, Michigan

Dale R. Romsos, (127) Department of Food Science and Human Nutrition, Michigan State University, East Lansing, Michigan

George Rouser, (225) Division of Neurosciences, City of Hope, National Medical Center, Duarte, California

Ann C. Sullivan, (143) Department of Biochemical Nutrition, Roche Research Center, Hoffman-La Roche, Inc., Nutley, New Jersey

Kenneth R. Warren, (87) Department of Cellular Physiology, Walter Reed Army Center, Walter Reed Army Institute of Research, Washington, D.C.

Lloyd A. Witting, (1) 3409 Dunes Lane, Denton, Texas

Preface

Over the last 20 years essentially every symposium dealing with the topic *Modification of Lipid Metabolism* has referred to atherosclerosis and hyperlipemia. The present symposium, held at the American Chemical Society Meeting in Atlantic City, New Jersey, September 10–11, 1974, was convened to demonstrate that constructive, progressive work has been done and is being done in other areas of lipid metabolism.

The chapter by Lloyd A. Witting is concerned with recent advances in the composition, structure, and functions of lipids in metabolic pathways. Our knowledge of the biosynthetic pathways for lipid synthesis has progressed to the point where the mode of synthesis of a new lipid may frequently be correctly predicted as soon as it is isolated and characterized. Emphasis is focused on the range and diversity encountered in common pathways in different species. Frequently, it is the unusual variation or block in a common reaction that offers the necessary insight into the manner in which the reaction is normally conducted.

The chapter by Joyce L. Beare-Rogers deals with a major problem for Canadian and European edible oil consumers and suppliers. After reports appeared that the consumption of erucic acid in rapeseed oil resulted in transitory fatty infiltration of the heart and residual cardiac necrosis and fibrosis in the male weanling rat, the composition of commercial rapeseed oil was drastically altered by genetic selection. The chapters by Michel Philippart and Norman S. Radin *et al.* discuss the genetic lipid storage diseases including diagnosis and treatment. Several methods of treatment are under active investigation, including the use of immobilized enzymes, organ transplants, and synthetic inhibitors. Viral modification of cell surface glycosphingolipids appears to be an important factor in contact inhibition of cell growth and division. Studies in this area, reviewed in the chapter by Peter H. Fishman and Roscoe O. Brady are vital to the understanding of the mode of action of oncogenic agents.

It is frequently stated that the nutritional problems in our affluent society are those associated with overconsumption. The chapters by Dale R. Romsos and Gilbert A. Leveille and Ann C. Sullivan refer to different approaches to the problem of obesity, dietary regulation of lipid storage and the use of a metabolic inhibitor to reduce lipid storage. After all the fad diets and quackery associated with the control of obesity, here are carefully controlled scientific studies of this all too common problem of concern to every fat chemist. The importance of perinatal nutrition is emphasized in the chapter by M. R. C. Greenwood. While malnutrition may reduce brain cell number, overnutrition increases adipose cell number. Most of our truly obese adults were apparently fat babies and have an excessive number of adipocytes in which to store fat.

The chapter by A. Saari Csallany and Roger I. Brooks reviews those factors in the environment that may effect tissue lipids and their metabolism. This is a rapidly developing area, the importance of which has only recently been realized.

The chapter by Roland C. Aloia and George Rouser reviews the phase transitions that have been observed in membranes and relates the effect of temperature changes on changes in lipids and proteins of membranes. This is of interest as it is related to growth and survival under adverse conditions.

When one considers how little was known about the pathways for lipid biosynthesis and their regulation as late as 1954, considerable progress has been made when only 20 years later it is possible to talk constructively about *Modification of Lipid Metabolism.*

The editors wish to acknowledge the cooperation of the contributors and the Illinois Agriculture Experiment Station for their support in preparation of the manuscript. A special thanks is extended to Ms. Vera Hodel and Stephanie Heard, who typed the manuscript.

Edward G. Perkins
Lloyd A. Witting

*Modification
of Lipid
Metabolism*

Recent Developments in Lipid
Biosynthetic Pathways

LLOYD A. WITTING

I. Introduction

Efforts to modify lipid metabolism presuppose extensive knowledge of the biosynthesis of lipids and the op-
eration of regulatory mechanisms. In the last 20 years,
such extensive information actually has been amassed. Not
only is it known how most lipids are synthesized in some
specific organism, but frequently an extensive literature
exists on the range and variations in pathways encountered
through many plant and animal phyla. Comparative biochemistry of this type often offers interesting insight into
the regulatory processes.

Some emphasis has been placed on the intensely interesting borderline area between lipid and carbohydrate
chemistry. The polyisoprenols form a novel bridge between
these fields. It is also a difficult problem as to whether
the glycolipids with long oligosaccharide chains should be
considered lipids or complex carbohydrates. For this
review, the discussion has been arbitrarily limited to
those compounds not containing more than 5 or 6 sugar residues.

After years of controversy, many of the problems associated with the complex interrelations between vitamin E,
biologically available selenium, sulfur amino acids, and
polyunsaturated fatty acids seem to have been resolved.
The biosynthesis of unsaturated fatty acids, while extensively investigated, still appears to require a breakthrough for its resolution.

II. Phospholipids

There have been several recent significant developments in the pathways for the synthesis of specific phospholipids including sphingomyelin, phosphatidylethanolamine,
diphosphatidylglycerol, and plasmalogens.

III. Sphingomyelin

Sribney and Kennedy (1958) described the reaction between a ceramide and CDP-choline to produce sphingomyelin.

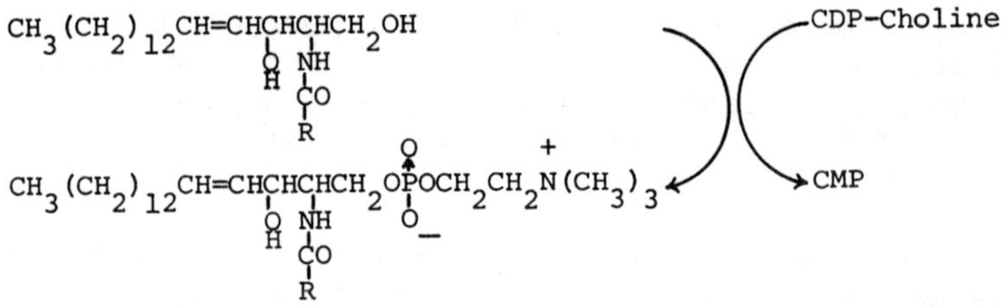

$$CH_3(CH_2)_{12}CH=CHCHCHCH_2OH$$

$$CH_3(CH_2)_{12}CH=CHCHCHCH_2OPOCH_2CH_2N(CH_3)_3$$

CDP-Choline

CMP

Unfortunately, this reaction proceeds best with the amides
of threo sphingosine and the naturally occurring sphingo-
myelins contain erythro sphingosine. Diringer *et al.*
(1972; Diringer and Koch, 1973) at Tubingen and Ullman and
Radin (1973; 1974) at Michigan have shown that sphingomyelin biosynthesis may proceed via a group transfer from
phosphatidylcholine to the erythro ceramide. This reaction
does not involve free CDP-choline, choline or phospho-
choline. The microsomal enzyme system found by Ullman and
Radin (1973; 1974) in mouse kidney, lung, liver, spleen,
and heart showed a preference for the ceramide-containing
palmitic acid, but also reacted with the ceramides containing lignoceric or nervonic acid.

$$C_{15}H_{29}\underset{\underset{\underset{R''}{CO}}{\overset{H}{\underset{|}{NH}}}}{\overset{|}{CHCHCH_2OH}}$$

$$C_{15}H_{29}CHCHCH_2\overset{O}{\underset{O_-}{\overset{\uparrow}{OPOCH_2CH_2N(CH_3)_3}}} \quad +$$

$$\begin{array}{l} CH_2OCOR \\ | \\ CHOCOR' \\ | \quad O \\ CH_2O\overset{\uparrow}{\underset{O_-}{P}}OCH_2CH_2N(CH_3)_3 \end{array} \quad +$$

$$\begin{array}{l} CH_2OCOR \\ | \\ CHOCOR' \\ | \\ CH_2OH \end{array}$$

IV. Bacterial Pathways

Bacterial pathways for the biosynthesis of several phospholipids have been shown to differ from the comparable mammalian pathways. While phosphatidylethanolamine is synthesized from diglyceride and CDP-ethanolamine in rat liver, the reaction in *E. coli* involves CDP-diglyceride and serine and requires decarboxylation of the intermediate phosphatidylserine (Raetz and Kennedy, 1972).

Phosphatidylglycerol appears to be synthesized via the same pathway in mammalian and bacterial systems, but the pathways to diphosphatidylglycerol, cardiolipin, may differ. In the first case, phosphatidylglycerol and CDP-diglyceride react to produce cardiolipin whereas *E. coli* condenses 2 molecules of phosphatidylglycerol to produce diphosphatidylglycerol and free glycerol (Hirschberg and Kennedy, 1972).

V. Glyceryl Ethers

Chimyl, batyl, and selachyl alcohols, the glyceryl ethers of the alcohols corresponding to palmitic, stearic, and oleic acids, have been known since the work of Tsujimoto and Toyamo (1922) on the liver oils of elasmobrach fishes, sharks, and rays. Similarly, the phospholipids of heart, brain, and several other tissues have been known to release fatty aldehydes upon acid hydrolysis since the

3

studies of Feulgen *et al.* (1929). Only recently have certain critical points in the biosynthesis of the alkyl glyceryl ethers and alk-1-enyl glycerol ethers been elucidated.

First, it was necessary to block the isomerization of dihydroxyacetone phosphate to glyceraldehyde phosphate by use of a suitable inhibitor (Wykle and Snyder, 1970). The key intermediate was then found to be 1-acyl dihydroxyacetone phosphate. In a reaction not yet completely characterized, Hajra (1970) found that a fatty alcohol replaces the acyl group. The oxygen (Snyder *et al.*, 1970) and both α-hydrogens (Wykle and Snyder, 1970) of the alcohol are retained in the ether, but one hydrogen from the triose carbon involved in the ester linkage is lost (Friedberg *et al.*, 1971; Friedberg and Heifetz, 1973). Reduction of the keto group, acylation, and dephosphorylation bring the molecule to a branch point which may lead either to a neutral lipid or to a phospholipid (Snyder, 1972). Desaturation of the ether takes place in the intact phospholipid (Blank *et al.*, 1972; Paltauf and Holasek, 1973).

Norton and Brotz (1963) reported that the galactosyl derivative of an alkyl, acyl glycerol occurs in mammalian brain. This compound is a myelin lipid and its synthesis (Wenger *et al.*, 1970) and degradation (Rao and Pieringer, 1970) have been described. Recently, it has been reported that the sulfated form of this ether lipid occurs in the testes. This lipid has been studied by Kornblatt *et al.* (1972; Knapp *et al.*, 1973) in Toronto and by Suzuki *et al.* (1973; Handa *et al.*, 1974) in Tokyo. The Japanese group refers to this compound as seminolipid. It has been shown that the sulfate group is transferred to the lipid from phosphoadenosylphosphosulfate, PAPS.

Kates has characterized 2 sulfated glyceryl ether derivatives in *Halobacterium cutirubrum* (Hancock and Kates, 1973; Kates and Deroo, 1973). In both cases, the phosphatidylglycerol sulfate and the glyceryl trihexoside sulfate, the lipids are diphytyl ethers. Phytol, 3,7,11,15-tetramethyl-hexadecanol, usually appears as a degradation product of chlorophyll. The biosynthetic pathways are not known, but reaction of PAPS with the phosphatidylglycerol would be anticipated. Similarly, the glycerol diether would be expected to react sequentially with UDP-Glc, GDP-Man, UDP-Gal, and PAPS.

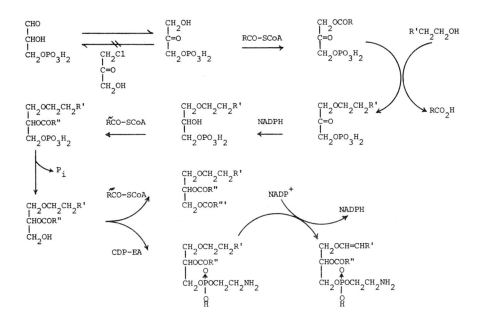

VI. Glycolipids

Lipid research is now going through a period of intense interest in glycolipids. This field may to some
extent be divided into three areas: relatively small glycolipids, oligosaccharides containing lipid, and the poly-
prenyl derivatives involved in the assembly of complex
materials such as glycoproteins, teichoic acids, lipopoly-
saccharides, and polysaccharides.

VII. Small Glycolipids

The small glycolipids are, in general, assembled via
glycosyl transferases from the appropriate sugar nucleo-
tides. Receptor molecules include hydroxy acids, diglycerides, and ceramides.

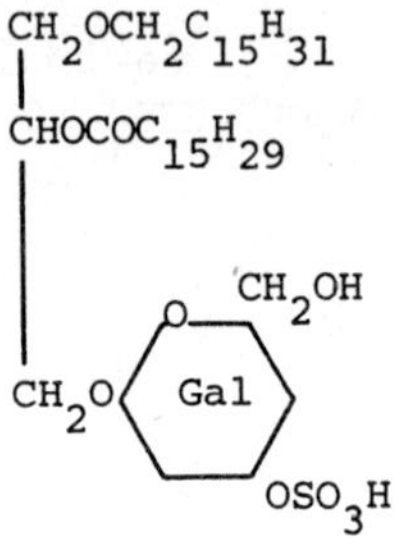

$CH_2OCH_2C_{15}H_{31}$
$CHOCOC_{15}H_{29}$

CH_2O ⟨ Gal ⟩

CH_2OH

OSO_3H

Yeasts and some fungi synthesize glycosides of hydroxy fatty acids such as the dirhamnoside of 3-hydroxy-decanoic acid in *Pseudomonas aeruginosa* (Jarvis and Johnson, 1949; Edwards and Hayashi, 1965) or the cellobioside of 15,16-dihydroxy-palmitic acid or 2,15,16-trihydroxy-palmitic acid

$CH_2OC_{20}H_{41}$
$CHOC_{20}H_{41}$

$CH_2OPOCH_2CHCH_2OSO_3H$

$CH_2OC_{20}H_{41}$
$CHOC_{20}H_{41}$
$CH_2OGlc-Man-Gal-OSO_3H$

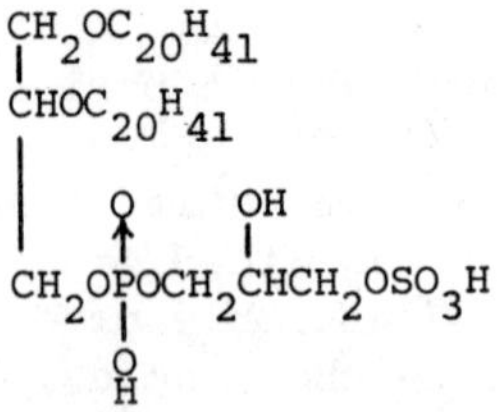

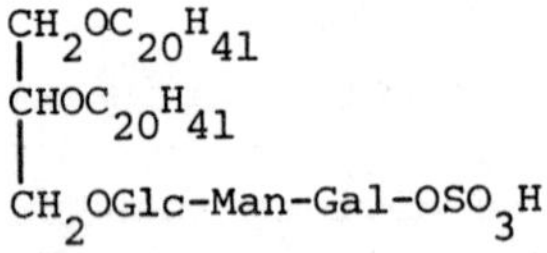

in the corn smut *Ustilago zeae* (Haskins, 1950; Lemieux, 1953). Synthesis of the dirhamnoside was described by

Burger *et al.* (1963). Steryl glycosides and acylated
steryl glycosides are synthesized by plants (Forsee *et al.*,
1974) and this subject has recently been reviewed by
Elbein *et al.* (1974).

In plants and gram-positive bacteria, the major glycolipids are usually diglycosyl diglycerides although longer
and shorter sugar chains are known (Shaw, 1970). Comparable
acidic lipids containing either glucuronic acid (Wilkinson,
1969) or galacturonic acid (Bergelson *et al.*, 1970) have
also been isolated. It is interesting to note that while
a variety of glycosyl diglycerides are known in bacteria,
members of the same genus contain the same glycolipid.
Several laboratories have shown that glycosyl diglycerides
are also found attached to phosphatidic acid (Smith, 1970)
or glyceryl phosphate (Peleg and Tietz, 1973). The synthesis (Pieringer, 1972) and function of these novel lipids
has recently been clarified by Pieringer and Ganfield
(1974).

Gram-positive bacteria have a complex cell wall which
contains small polymers known as teichoic acids. Various
teichoic acid structures have been identified including
poly(glyceryl phosphate) and polymers containing glyceryl
phosphate alternating with a hexose or hexosamine or the
corresponding sugar phosphates. Pieringer and Ganfield
(1974) have isolated the phosphoglycolipid with teichoic
acid fragments attached and suggest that the linkage is between a phosphate from the teichoic acid and a hydroxyl
group of a lipid bound glucose. An interesting cross-
linking of the lipid membrane and cell wall results.

Ceramides with oligosaccharide chains of various
lengths are widely distributed, but this discussion will
consider only the more common mammalian compounds with 5 or
fewer sugar residues. Synthesis proceeds by a progressive
buildup of the linear oligosaccharide chain on the ceramide
by the appropriate glycosyl transferases and becomes complicated only when the sequence of addition of sialic acid
units must be considered (Svennerholm, 1970; Wiegandt, 1971;
Ramsey and Nicholas, 1972; Suzuki, 1972; Bowen *et al.*, 1974;
Burton, 1974). This area has been intensively studied
since a number of lipid storage diseases are known related
to genetic errors affecting the degradation of these
glycosphingolipids.

Galactosyl ceramide and the corresponding sialic acid derivative (Siddiqui and McCluer, 1968) and sulfate are well-known as brain lipids and the digalactosyl ceramide (Adams and Grey, 1970) occurs in kidney lipids. The other major glycosphingolipids, of which there are at least 5 series of compounds, are derived from lactosyl ceramide, GalGlcCer. The sulfate of lactosyl ceramide appears in kidney (Martensson, 1963; Martensson, 1966) and the sialic acid derivative is rather widely distributed throughout the tissues.

To some extent, the variations in the oligosaccharide chains are related to the area in which the lipids are found. Globosides, GalNAcβ1-3Galα1-4Galβ1-4GlcCer, (Hakomori et al., 1971; Laine et al., 1972) and the corresponding shorter oligosaccharides are associated with bone marrow, spleen, and blood elements. The isomeric compound, GalNAcβ1-3Galα1-3Galβ1-4GlcCer, has been called cytolipin R, although isogloboside might be a more appropriate designation, has been found in rat kidney (Siddiqui et al., 1972). Ganglio-N-tetraose, Galβ1-3GalNAcβ1-4Galβ1-4Glc, is the basic oligosaccharide of the brain gangliosides. The monosialo derivative of this ceramide tetrasaccharide is frequently referred to as Ganglioside G_{M1}, whereas Gangliosides G_{M2} and G_{M3} are the corresponding monosialo derivatives of ceramide ganglio-N-triose and lactosyl ceramide, respectively. Lactosyl ceramide is also a precursor to the N-tetraose series found in extraneural

gangliosides and thus may be described as a member of
either or both sets of gangliosides.

The sugar sequences found to occur in the extraneural
gangliosides and blood group active lipids were previously
shown to occur in oligosaccharides in milk (Kuhn and Baer,
1956; Kuhn and Gauhe, 1962; Ginsburg, 1972), and the
nomenclature is based on these compounds, lacto-N-tetraose
Galβ1-3GlcNAcβ1-3Galβ1-4Glc and lacto-N-neotetraose Galβ1-
4GlcNAcβ1-3Galβ1-4Glc. Wiegandt (1973) has stated that
most of the extraneural gangliosides are based on the
lacto-N-neotetraose structure. The major ganglioside isolated from human erythrocytes by Wherrett (1973), NANA 2-3
Galβ1-4GlcNAcβ1-3Galβ1-4GlcCer, corresponds to one of the
monosialo gangliosides isolated by Wiegandt (1973) from
human and bovine spleen. Ceramide lacto-N-neotetraose has
been referred to as paragloboside or as an asialoganglio-
side (Wherrett, 1973).

Type 1 structures (Ginsburg, 1972) responsible for
H, A, B, Le[a] and Le[b] specificities have the Galβ1-3GlcNAc
sequence of lacto-N-tetraose, while Type 2 structures have
the Galβ1-4GlcNAc sequence of lacto-N-neotetraose. Structures with H, A, B, and Le[b] specificity have fucose attached to the galactose residue and the Le[a] and Le[b] specific structures have fucose attached to the GlcNAc unit.
A and B specific structures also have GalNAc and Gal,
respectively, attached to the galactose. There has been
intense interest in compounds of this type, most of which
fall into the class described below as complex carbohydrates containing lipid.

The five major series of ceramide polyhexosides are
defined by the N-tetraoses, but several of the ceramide
pentasaccharides are relatively important. The Forssman
hapten, GalNAcα1-3Globo-N-tetraosyl ceramide, found in
equine spleen (Siddiqui and Hakomori, 1971) has been reported to be the major glycolipid in caprine erythrocytes
(Taketomi and Kawamura, 1972) and also occurs in canine
intestine (Vance et al., 1966). Two separate glycosyl
transferases are involved in the sequential addition of
GalNAc units to ceramide trihexoside and globoside to form
this ceramide pentahexoside (Ishibashi et al., 1974;
Kijimoto et al., 1974). Galactosyl lacto-N-tetraosyl
ceramide has been described as the major glycolipid in
rabbit erythrocytes (Eto et al., 1968). Galactosyl
ganglio-N-tetraosyl ceramide has been reported in the

gangliosides of several species (Svennerholm et al., 1973).
Wiegandt has reported that fucosyl ganglio-N-teraosyl
ceramide occurs in bovine liver gangliosides (Wiegandt,
1974).

It will be quite interesting to see why such species
differences exist and how the special uses of the various
glycosphingolipids are determined by the tetrasaccharide
sequence. Two particularly important aspects of glyco-
sphingolipid metabolism, genetic lipid storage disease,
and modification of cell surface lipids by viruses, are
considered elsewhere in this volume.

VIII. Complex Carbohydrates Containing Lipid

Blood group activity is presumably determined largely
by certain glycoproteins (Ginsburg, 1972), but the critical
oligosaccharide sequences also appear linked to ceramides.
Compounds of this type containing 12-14 sugar residues
have been described by Hakomori et al. (1972). Many of
these compounds are soluble in lipid solvents such as
chloroform-methanol and may be eluted from silicic acid
columns with chloroform-methanol-acetone-water mixtures.
The sequences of the sugars are genetically determined and
the critical sequences are at a distance from the ceramide
unit. These compounds are basically a problem for the
carbohydrate chemist and, therefore, will not be considered
further here.

IX. Polyisoprenols

Instead of transferring sugar residues one by one
from the appropriate nucleotide derivatives to the acceptor
molecule, it is conceivable that the oligosaccharide could
be built up on a carrier and transferred intact to the acceptor. Reactions of this type are known to occur and in
such reactions, the intermediate carrier is a derivative
of a polyisoprenoid alcohol.

The all-trans-nonaprenyl alcohol, solanesol, was isolated from tobacco by Rowland, Latimer, and Giles (1956).
Between 1963 and 1967, somewhat similar alcohols containing 6-22 isoprenoid units were isolated from various
sources. These compounds are synthesized by the addition
of cis isoprenoid units from isopentenyl pyrophosphate to

either all-*trans*-farnesyl pyrophosphate or all-*trans*-geranylgeranyl pyrophosphate. The configuration of the terminal isoprene units in the $C_{30}-C_{45}$ compounds from birch wood (Wellburn and Hemming, 1966) and the $C_{50}-C_{65}$ alcohols from bacteria (Gough *et al.*, 1970) correspond to the elongation of all-*trans*-geranylgeraniol. Dolichols, the $C_{70}-C_{90}$ compounds from yeast (Dunphy *et al.*, 1966) and the $C_{85}-C_{110}$ compounds from mammals (Dunphy *et al.*, 1967), are based on farnesol, but have a saturated isoprene unit at the hydroxyl end of the molecule. Other partially hydrogenated structures are also known with hexahydropolyisoprenols in the $C_{95}-C_{115}$ range in *Aspergilus* (Butterworth *et al.*, 1966) and an octahydroheptaisoprenol in *Mycobacterium smegmatis* (Tayama *et al.*, 1973). These polyisoprenols occur in groups of similar chain length although one chain length is usually predominant. Minor variations in the number of *cis* double bonds also appear to be prevalent.

The active form of the polyisoprenol is the phosphorylated derivative. These molecules act as carriers in at least 3 types of reactions.

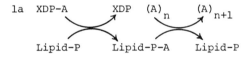

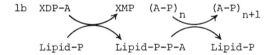

Reactions of type la involve the simple transfer of some material, A, from the appropriate nucleotide derivative, XDP-A, to a growing polymer, $(A)_n$ via the polyisoprenol phosphate, Lipid-P-A. An example of this type of reaction would be the transfer of mannose units from GDP-Man to mannan (Scher and Lennarz, 1969; Lahav *et al.*, 1969). Type lb reactions involve transfer of a phosphorylated unit to a growing polymer. In this case, the intermediate is a polyisoprenol pyrophosphate derivative, Lipid-P-P-A, but the polyisoprenol phosphate is regenerated since the second phosphate is transferred as part of the monomer unit. An example of this type of reaction is the formation of a teichoic acid, such as (glycerol phosphate)$_n$ (Anderson et al., 1972) or (GlcNAc-P)$_n$ (Watkinson et al., 1971).

Reactions of Type 2 involve assembly of 2 different units on the lipid carrier prior to transfer of both to the growing polymer. An alternating structure of the type common in teichoic acids results. One or both units may be phosphorylated as in (Glycerol-P-Glc)$_n$ (Burger and Glaser, 1966) or (Glycerol-P-NAcGlc-P)$_n$ (Hancock and Baddiley, 1972).

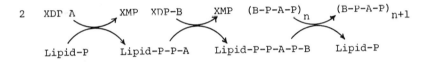

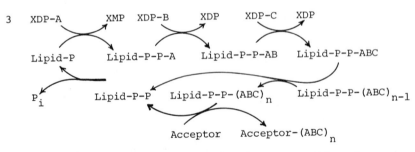

The third type of reaction involves assembly of a complex monomer unit on a polyisoprenol derivative and polymerization of these monomer units on a carrier molecule of polyisoprenol prior to transfer to the acceptor. An example is the assembly of the O-antigen, $\binom{Abe}{Man}$-Rha-Gal)$_n$, which becomes part of a lipopolysaccharide (Osborn, 1966). Polyisoprenol pyrophosphate is a product of the reaction and a specific phosphatase is required to regenerate the monophosphate. The units assembled on the lipid carrier are in some cases more complicated than the examples cited and are not limited to carbohydrates. In S. aureus, for instance, the repeating unit of the cell wall, peptidoglycan, consists of N-acetylglucosamine, N-acetylmuraminic acid, and a decapeptide (Strominger et al., 1972). Similarly, the products are not restricted to exotic bacterial materials and include mammalian glycoproteins and polysaccharides. This area has recently been reviewed by Hemming (1974).

X. Fatty Acids

Involvement of 2 multienzyme complexes, acetyl-CoA-carboxylase and fatty acid synthetase, in fatty acid biosynthesis has presented the enzymologist with a variety of difficult problems. This area has been reviewed by Volpe and Vagelos (1973) and Vagelos (1974). Only relatively simple fatty acids of limited chain length appear to be produced via this pathway. In *E. coli*, the activity of the condensing enzymes decreases with increasing fatty acid chain length such that the major saturated end product is palmitic acid (Greenspan *et al.*, 1970). In gram-negative bacteria, the action of β-hydroxyl decanoyl thioester dehydrase to produce *cis*-Δ^3-decanoate in place of *trans*-Δ^2-decanoate results in "anaerobic" synthesis of palmitoleic acid, Δ^9 16:1ω7, and vaccenic acid Δ^{11}-18:1ω7 in addition to palmitate (Erwin and Bloch, 1964; Kaas *et al.*, 1967; Bloch, 1969). For gram-positive bacteria, the corresponding end products are the C_{15}-C_{17} iso and anteiso branched chain fatty acids (Lynen, 1972). The mammalian fatty acid synthetase also produces mainly palmitic acid, but this may be related to the activity of a specific thioesterase (Barnes and Wakil, 1968).

Problems of current interest are oxygen dependent desaturation, elongation of fatty acids beyond the C_{16} level, hydroxylation and ether formation.

XI. Unsaturated Fatty Acid Biosynthesis

There has been considerable interest in the synthesis of fatty acids containing more than one double bond. It is generally stated (Stumpf *et al.*, 1972) that most higher plants insert additional double bonds only between the existing double bonds and the terminal methyl group, while animals add additional double bonds only between the existing double bonds and the carboxyl group. The limitations of this highly oversimplified statement have been the subject of numerous investigations.

It is convenient to use 2 separate systems for designating the position of the double bonds. Oleic acid and linoleic acid are Δ^9-18:1 and $\Delta^{9,12}$-18:2, respectively, when the positions of the double bonds are numbered from the carboxyl group and 18:1ω9 and 18:2ω6, respectively, when numbered from the terminal methyl group. The omega nomenclature is restricted to use with fatty acids containing only methylene interrupted double bonds, $CH_3(CH_2)_x$ $(CH=CHCH_2)_n(CH_2)_yCOH$, since otherwise the position of the final double bond is unspecified. The reasons for the use of these numbering systems will become evident in the following discussion.

The synthesis of most of the known simple polyunsaturated fatty acids, PUFA, can be explained in terms of 3 "plant" desaturase activities introducing double bonds at the ω9, ω6, and ω3 positions and 4 "animal" desaturase activities introducing double bonds at the Δ^4, Δ^5, Δ^6, and Δ^9 positions as diagrammed in Figure 1.

The series of C_{16} PUFA occurring in algae and elsewhere as noted below emphasize the omega orientation of the plant desaturase activities. Similarly, the odd chain length fatty acids chemically synthesized by Schlenk (1970) are also appropriate substrates for the animal desaturase activities and emphasize the delta orientation in double bond production.

$\Delta^{9,12}$ 17:2ω5 $\longrightarrow \Delta^{6,9,12}$ 17:3ω5 $\longrightarrow \Delta^{8,11,14}$ 19:3ω5 $\longrightarrow \Delta^{5,8,11,14}$ 19:4ω5

$\Delta^{9,12}$ 19:2ω7 $\longrightarrow \Delta^{6,9,12}$ 19:3ω5 $\longrightarrow \Delta^{8,11,14}$ 21:3ω7 $\longrightarrow \Delta^{5,8,11,14}$ 21:4ω7

Plant Desaturase Activities, ω9, ω6 and ω3

16:0 → Δ^7 16:1ω9 → $\Delta^{7,10}$ 16:2ω6 → $\Delta^{7,10,13}$ 16:3ω3

18:0 → Δ^9 18:1ω9 → $\Delta^{9,12}$ 18:2ω6 → $\Delta^{9,12,15}$ 18:3ω3

Animal Desaturase Activities

16:0 → Δ^9 16:1ω7 → Δ^6 $\Delta^{6,9}$ 16:2ω7 → $\Delta^{8,11}$ 18:2ω7 → Δ^5 $\Delta^{5,8,11}$ 18:3ω7 → $\Delta^{7,10,13}$ 20:3ω7 → Δ^4 $\Delta^{4,7,10,13}$ 20:4ω7

18:0 → Δ^9 18:1ω9 → $\Delta^{6,9}$ 18:2ω9 → $\Delta^{8,11}$ 20:2ω9 → $\Delta^{5,8,11}$ 20:3ω9 → $\Delta^{7,10,13}$ 22:3ω9 → $\Delta^{4,7,10,13}$ 22:4ω9

$\Delta^{9,12}$ 18:2ω6 → $\Delta^{6,9,12}$ 18:3ω6 → $\Delta^{8,11,14}$ 20:3ω6 → $\Delta^{5,8,11,14}$ 20:4ω6 → $\Delta^{7,10,13,16}$ 22:4ω6 → $\Delta^{4,7,10,13,16}$ 22:5ω6

$\Delta^{9,12,15}$ 18:3ω3 → $\Delta^{6,9,12,15}$ 18:4ω3 → $\Delta^{8,11,14,17}$ 20:4ω3 → $\Delta^{5,8,11,14,17}$ 20:5ω3 → $\Delta^{7,10,13,16,19}$ 22:5ω3 → $\Delta^{4,7,10,13,16,19}$ 22:6ω3

Fig. 1. Progressive desaturation of unsaturated fatty acids of plant origin by plant and animal desaturases.

Plant desaturases appear to act only in a sequential manner. The introduction of an $\omega 6$ double bond requires the presence of a double bond in the $\omega 9$ position and introduction of an $\omega 3$ double bond requires double bonds in the $\omega 9$ and $\omega 6$ positions. Animal desaturases also usually act in a sequential manner alternating with chain elongation. Introduction of a Δ^5 double bond in a fatty acid with a Δ^6 double bond must be preceded by chain elongation as must the introduction of a Δ^4 double bond in a fatty acid containing a Δ^5 double bond. As noted below, Δ^4, Δ^5, and Δ^6 monoenoic fatty acids may be produced from saturated fatty acids and double bonds may be introduced in these positions in fatty acids acted upon by the omega desaturases.

Various published diagrams, such as that of Gurr and James (1971) used to describe the interconversions of PUFA, freely illustrate reactions which would require desaturases acting at the Δ^7, Δ^8, and Δ^{10} positions. Gurr (1974), however, in tabulating desaturase activities suggests that unsaturation is *not* directly introduced into these locations. Sprecher (1971) has shown that in the rat $\Delta^{5,8,11}$ 18:3ω7 and $\Delta^{7,10,13}$ 20:3ω7 are converted to $\Delta^{4,7,10,13}$ 20:4ω7, but the reaction proceeds very poorly with $\Delta^{10,13}$ 20:2ω7. The Δ^7 double bond must be introduced as a Δ^5 double bond at the C_{18} level, $\Delta^{10,13}$ 20:2ω7 $\rightarrow$ $\Delta^{8,11}$ 18:2ω7 $\rightarrow$ $\Delta^{5,8,11}$ 18:3ω7 $\rightarrow$ $\Delta^{7,10,13}$ 20:3ω7. The importance of retroconversion, the shortening of a PUFA by 2 carbons, has only been fully appreciated in the last few years. For instance, the investigators who discovered a novel fatty acid, $\Delta^{3,6,9,12,15}$ 18:5ω3, in cultured dynoflagellates immediately considered this possibility and showed that the compound arose from retroconversion of $\Delta^{5,8,11,14,17}$ 20:5ω3 (Joseph, 1974).

The desaturase situation is not entirely clear at the monoenoic acid level, but the evidence for the occurrence of a "plant" $\omega 9$ desaturase activity is good. Hilditch (1940) noted that palmitoleic acid, Δ^9 16:1ω7, was originally named physetoleic acid by Hofstadter who isolated the fatty acid from the head oil of the sperm whale in 1854. Subsequent isolations were from seal oil (1898) and cod liver oil (1906). Palmitoleic acid is most abundant in aquatic species and higher animals and is rarely presented at levels over 1% in the fats of higher plants. Hypogaeic acid, Δ^7 16:1ω9, has been reported in a few seed oils (Groessman and Scheren, 1855; Klenk and Steinbach, 1959). Oleic acid, Δ^9 18:1ω9, could be produced by either a Δ^9 or an $\omega 9$ desaturase.

Green algae are the major source of C_{16} PUFA (Erwin, 1973). In *Chlorella vulgaris* Δ^7 16:1ω9 and Δ^9 16:1ω7 are synthesized by separate enzymes and the enzyme introducing the ω9 (Δ^7) bond in 16:0 was not active on 18:0 (Brett *et al.*, 1971). Except in an aberrant pathway in diatoms (Klenk and Eberhagen, 1962), only the Δ^7 16:1ω9 is converted to PUFA. James has commented on this point (James, 1972). Stearns (1970) found that soybean oil contains traces of Δ^7 16:1ω9 and $\Delta^{7,10}$ 16:2ω6. These fatty acids were also found in 4 of 5 species of *Ranunculus* (Spencer *et al.*, 1970), *Ginkgo biloba* leaves, and cashew nuts (Gellerman and Schlenk, 1968). Ferns (Radunz, 1967) and moss lipids (Anderson *et al.*, 1972; Gellerman and Schlenk, 1964) have also been reported to contain relatively large quantities of $\Delta^{7,10,13}$ 16:1ω3. Stumpf's group (Jacobson *et al.*, 1973a; 1973b) has presented evidence that in a higher plant, spinach, linolenic acid, $\Delta^{9,12,15}$ 18:3ω3, arises from elongation of $\Delta^{7,10,13}$ 16:1ω3 rather than from desaturation of linoleic acid, $\Delta^{9,12}$ 18:2ω6. This might be interpreted as an ω6 desaturase activity acting on either Δ^7 16:1ω9 or Δ^9 18:1ω9, but an ω3 desaturase activity that cannot utilize the C_{18} acid as a substrate.

A number of investigators have presented data relevant to the appearance of the various desaturase activities at different stages of the evolutionary process. In the animal kingdom, until very recently, the data were derived from a few protozoa and a few vertebrates. Much of our information on higher animals is based on investigations, not directly of biosynthetic pathways, but rather of requirements for "essential" fatty acids. For instance, the rat and rainbow trout (Castell *et al.*, 1972a; 1972b) on fat-free diets accumulate eicosatrienoic acids, 20:3ω9 and 20:3ω7, and show evidence of a nutritional deficiency. In the rat, the essential fatty acid requirement is met by a source of ω6 PUFA, while the fish requires a source of ω3 PUFA and does not respond to ω6 PUFA (Sinnhuber *et al.*, 1972). A few insects also seem to require "essential" fatty acids (Earle *et al.*, 1967). Linoleic acid is the usual ω6 "essential" fatty acid, but other fatty acids also have this activity.

Klenk (1965) has shown that $\Delta^{7,10}$ 16:2ω6 is converted to linoleic acid by the rat. Sprecher (1968) confirmed this observation and showed that $\Delta^{5,8}$ 14:2ω6 is a relatively poor precursor for linoleic acid in the rat and $\Delta^{3,6}$ 12:2ω6 and Δ^4 10:1ω6 are not utilized for this pur-

pose. The chicken, however, appears to be able to synthesize linoleate from cis-Δ^2 18:1ω6 (Reiser et $al.$, 1962).
Gurr et $al.$ (1972) found that linoleic acid can be produced
in good yield from Δ^{12} 18:1ω6 by the goat, hen, and pig and
in poor yield by the mouse and rabbit, while the rat and
hamster are unable to effect this conversion.

The deficiency approach fails to identify those organisms that may have only "animal" desaturase activities,
but do not require PUFA-containing double bonds in positions acted upon only by "plant" desaturases. Protozoa
grown on strictly fat-free media synthesize 18:2ω6 and
18:3ω6, but apparently have little if any ω3 PUFA (Erwin,
1973; Korn et $al.$, 1965). Recently, evidence was presented
suggesting that the pulmonate snail, a mollusc, is able to
synthesize 18:2ω6, but not ω3 PUFA (Van Der Horst, 1973).
It seems possible that the ω6 desaturase activity, but not
the ω3 desaturase activity, may be present in many lower
animals.

It is much easier to obtain information on fatty acid
biosynthesis in photoauxotrophic species than in heterotrophic organisms. All of the plant phyla have been rather
extensively investigated and each appears to contain members possessing one or more of the "animal" desaturase
activities.

Although most bacteria synthesize monoenoic fatty
acids by the "anaerobic" pathway (Erwin and Bloch, 1964;
Kass et $al.$, 1967; Bloch, 1969), a number of $Bacilli$ synthesize Δ^5 16:1 and Δ^5 18:1 by an oxygen dependent mechanism (Fulco et $al.$, 1964; Fulco, 1967; Kaneda, 1971; Fulco,
1969a) and a few synthesize mixtures of the Δ^8, Δ^9, and Δ^{10}
isomers of hexadecenoic acid (Fulco, 1969a; Dart and Kaneda,
1970). Both desaturase activities are present in $B.$ $lichen$-
$formis$ and $\Delta^{5,10}$ 16:2 is produced (Fulco, 1969b; Fulco,
1970). Similar fatty acids containing isolated cis-Δ^5
double bonds are found in a slime mold (Davidoff and Korn,
1962; Davidoff and Korn, 1963) a sponge (Jefferts et $al.$,
1974), algae (Jamieson and Reid, 1972), a number of higher
plants (Spencer et $al.$, 1969; Kleiman et $al.$, 1972; Smith
et $al.$, 1968; Smith et $al.$, 1969; Schlenk and Gellerman,
1965; Powell et $al.$, 1967; Smith et $al.$, 1960; Ito et $al.$,
1963; Takagi, 1964; Bagby et $al.$, 1961), and possibly in
a variety of marine animals (Ackman and Hooper, 1973a).

Kenyon (1972a) and Kenyon et $al.$ (1972b) have analyzed

SOURCES OF Δ^5 FATTY ACIDS

Δ^5 16:1

    Bacilli (62,67,107)

    Carlina corymbosa (186)

    Chenopodiaceae cp (114)

$\Delta^{5,9}$ 16:1

    Dictyostelium discoideum
    (39,40)

$\Delta^{5,10}$ 16:1

    Bacillus lichenformis (64,65)

Δ^5 18:1

    Bacillus megaterium (62)

    Caltha palustris (182)

    Carlina corymbosa (186)

    Chenopodiaceae sp (114)

$\Delta^{5,9}$ 18:2

    Dictyostelium discoideum
    (39,40)

    Chenopodiaceae sp (114)

    Teucrium depressum (180)

$\Delta^{5,11}$ 18:2

    Dictyostelium discoideum
    (39,40)

    Ginkgo biloba (171)

$\Delta^{5,9,12}$ 18:3

    Chenopodiaceae sp (114)

    Xeranthenum annuum (154)

Δ^5 20:1

    Caltha palustris (182)

    Limnanthes douglasii (179)

$\Delta^{5,11}$ 20:2

    Ginkgo biloba (171)

    Molluscs and Crustaceans
    (?) (1)

$\Delta^{5,11,14}$

    Ascophyllium nodosum (100)

    Caltha palustris (182)

    Podocarpus nagi (94,201)

$\Delta^{5,11,14,17}$ 20:4

    Caltha palustris (182)

    Ginkgo biloba (171)

Δ^5 22:1

    Limnanthes douglasii (179)

$\Delta^{5,13}$ 22:2

    Limnanthes douglasii (9)

    Molluscs and Crustaceans
    (?) (1)

$\Delta^{5,9}$ 26:2

    Microciona prolifera (102)

$\Delta^{5,9,19}$ 26:3

    Microciona prolifera (102)

the fatty acids from a large number of filamentous and unicellular blue-green algae. Four metabolic groups were apparent which contained various combinations of the Δ^6, $\omega 6$, and $\omega 3$ desaturase activities in addition to the Δ^9 or $\omega 9$ activity. 1) none, 2) $\omega 6 + \omega 3$, 3) $\omega 6 + \Delta^6$, and 4) $\omega 6 + \omega 3 + \Delta^6$. The most highly unsaturated fatty acid in each group was therefore 1) $18:1\omega 9$, 2) $18:3\omega 3$, 3) $18:3\omega 6$ and 4) $18:4\omega 3$.

A somewhat comparable distribution of desaturase activities has been found in higher plants of the order *Umbelliferae*. The isolated Δ^6 double bond appears in petroselenic acid, Δ^6 $18:1\omega 12$, the predominant fatty acid in the families *Umbelliferae* and *Aralaceae* (Spencer *et al.*, (1971). Both petroselenic and oleic acids may occur in the same plant. Some species of *Liliaceae* contain $\Delta^{6,9,12}$ $18:3\omega 6$ (Morice, 1967) and *Echium rubrum* seed oil (Miller *et al.*, 1968) contains 34% $\Delta^{9,12,15}$ $18:3\omega 3$, 14% $\Delta^{6,9,12}$ $18:3\omega 6$, and 15% $\Delta^{6,9,12,15}$ $18:4\omega 3$. This tetraene also occurs in other members of the family *Boraginaceae* (Wagner and Konig, 1963; Craig and Bhatty, 1964; Smith *et al.*, 1964; Kleiman *et al.*, 1964; Jamieson and Reid, 1969). *Anemone cylindrica* (Spencer *et al.*, 1970) is unusual in having a level (19%) of $\Delta^{6,9,12}$ $18:3\omega 6$ comparable to many *Boraginaceae*.

Diatoms contain the Δ^6 desaturase activity, but it is combined with an aberrant pathway producing $\Delta^{9,12}$ $16:2\omega 4$ (Davidoff and Korn, 1963), $\Delta^{6,9,12}$ $16:3\omega 4$, and $\Delta^{6,9,12,15}$ $16:4\omega 1$ (Klenk and Eberhagen, 1962).

Both the Δ^6 and Δ^5 desaturase activities are found in green unicellular biflagellates which also have $\omega 6$ activity and arachidonic acid, $\Delta^{5,8,11,14}$ $20:4\omega 6$ is produced (Erwin, 1973). Red algae also contain $\omega 3$ activity and produce $\Delta^{5,8,11,14,17}$ $20:5\omega 3$ (Klenk *et al.*, 1963). *Phycomycetes* and *Ascomycetes* are usually distinguished from each other by their content of $18:3\omega 6$ and $18:3\omega 3$, respectively (Shaw, 1966). Many *Phycomycetes* also contain arachidonic acid (Erwin, 1973) and, therefore, also have Δ^5 desaturase activity. Mosses and ferns also contain Δ^5 and Δ^6 desaturase activities and produce $20:4\omega 6$ and $20:5\omega 3$ (Anderson *et al.*, 1972; Gellerman and Schlenk, 1964).

Desaturase activity of the Δ^4 type is apparently very rare in plants, although a few Δ^4 monoenoic acids are found in *Lauraccae* (Hopkins *et al.*, 1966). The Δ^4 activity is

20

combined with $\omega 9$, $\omega 6$, and $\omega 3$ activity in unicellular green algae to produce $\Delta^{4,7,10,13}$ 16:4ω3 (Korn, 1964). Both photosynthetic and heterotrophic dynoflagellates have been reported to synthesize $\Delta^{4,7,10,13,16,19}$ 22:6ω3 (Harrington et al., 1970).

Nature obviously does not strictly adhere to the artificial "plant" versus "animal" classification of desaturase activities. As more information becomes available on the lower animals, it is probable that a relatively coherent pattern of distribution will become apparent. Such research, however, will be impeded by the complications imposed by "essential" fatty acid requirements.

The mechanism of fatty acid desaturation has been reviewed by Gurr (1974) and Fulco (1974). Since the pioneering work of Bloomfield and Bloch (1960), a number of cell-free systems have been developed for studying the desaturation reaction and several of these systems have been solubilized. In each case, O_2 and a reduced pyridine nucleotide are required for double bond formation. Progress has been made in elucidating the electron transport system involved in the desaturation, but not in isolation of oxygenated intermediates. The rat microsomal stearate desaturase appears to involve at least 4 proteins (Oshino, 1972a; Oshino and Sato, 1972b).

The activated form of the fatty acid varies according to the system under study. Acyl-CoA derivatives are utilized by particulate desaturases from various bacteria, some yeasts, fungi and algae, and animal microsomes. Particular attention has recently been focused on the desaturation of oleate to linoleate in intact phospholipid (Gurr et al., 1969; Baker and Lynen, 1971; Pugh and Kates, 1973; Talamo et al., 1973).

Lyman et al. (1969; 1970) have presented data suggesting that feeding ethionine to the rat interferes with stearate desaturation and conversion of linoleate to arachidonate in vivo and in vitro. Vesicular dilatation of the hepatic endoplasmic reticulum occurs soon after feeding the hepatotoxin. The results observed on measurement of apparent desaturase activity were related, at least in part, to the increased susceptibility of the microsomes to damage during isolation and could be largely avoided by the addition of appropriate protective agents during processing of the tissue (Witting, 1973). This is consistent with the failure to observe decreased levels of unsaturated

fatty acids in the livers of the rats fed ethionine (Lyman
et al., 1969; Lyman et al., 1970).

XII. Fatty Acid Elongation and Hydroxylation

Modification of fatty acid structure has recently
been reviewed by Fulco (1974). Fatty acid chain elongation beyond palmitate is frequently associated with desaturation and is separated from the pathway involving the
fatty acid synthetase system. Mention has already been
made of the alternating desaturation and elongation steps
in PUFA biosynthesis on the "animal" pathway which occurs
in the endoplasmic reticulum.

The biological membrane is a dynamic structure and
reference is made to the "fluid" membrane. If the fatty
acid methyl esters are considered somewhat analogous to
the glyceryl linked fatty acids, it is interesting to note
that the melting points (Deuel, 1951) of the 16:0, 18:0,
20:0, 22:0, and 24:0 esters are 31°, 39°, 47°, 53°, and
58°C, respectively. The melting points of the corresponding free acids are approximately 30° higher. Introduction
of one relatively centrally located double bond lowers the
melting point significantly (24:1ω9, free acid, m.p. 43°).
Very long chain saturated and monoenoic fatty acids are
usually restricted to sphingolipids, particularly glycosphingolipids, and are often hydroxylated at the α-posi-
tion. The conspicuous exception to this generality is
in the waxes and surface lipids. This is an area of lipid
research in which there has been dramatic recent progress.

Waxes are usually thought of as water repellent outer
surface coatings, but may also be used for energy storage
or as a structural material (beeswax) and it has been suggested that they be involved in echolocation and in regulation of buoyancy in benthic species. Copepods collected
at a depth of 2500 meters not only contained high levels
of lipids, but very high percentages (20-90%) of the total
lipid was wax ester (Benson et al., 1972). In addition
to simple esters, waxes may also contain hydrocarbons,
hydroxy acids, alkane diols, ketones, diketones, secondary
alcohols, etc. Beeswax (Tulloch, 1970), for instance,
contains 16% hydrocarbons (C_{27}, C_{29}, C_{31}, C_{33}), 31% alcohols (C_{26}, C_{28}, C_{30}, C_{32}), 31% acids (C_{16}, C_{24}), 13% hydroxy acids (C_{16}, C_{24}), and 3% alkane diols (C_{24}, C_{26}, C_{28},
C_{30}). The component present at the highest level in each

series has been underlined. It is to be noted that the
diols are of the $\alpha,\omega-1$ type and the fatty acids are hydroxylated at the $\omega-1$ position. Several systems are known for
α-hydroxylation, but hydroxylation at more distant points
is usually attributed to a mixed function oxidase type
system (Fulco, 1974).

When the fatty acids, hydroxy acids, and primary
alcohols contain an even number of carbon atoms, the hydrocarbons have an odd chain length. Ketones and secondar-
y alcohols, when present, tend to have centrally located
functional groups ($C_{15}H_{31}COC_{15}H_{31}$), although 2-4 isomers
may be present ($C_{10}H_{21}CH(OH)C_{16}H_{33}$, $C_{11}H_{23}CH(OH)C_{15}H_{31}$,
$C_{12}H_{25}CH(OH)C_{14}H_{29}$, and $C_{13}H_{27}CH(OH)C_{13}H_{27}$) as in grass-
hoppers (Blomquist et al., 1972). A head to head conden-
sation of fatty acids was suggested to occur with the loss
of one of the carboxyl groups (Albro and Dittmer, 1970).
This pathway would seem to be supported by the occurrence
of hydrocarbons with iso and/or anteiso branching at both
ends of the molecule in gram-positive bacteria (Tornabene
and Markey, 1971). Kolattukudy et al. (1972a; 1972b);
Buckner and Kolattukudy, 1973) have shown that in plants
palmitate leaves the fatty acid synthetase complex and is
elongated further via malonyl-CoA by the endoplasmic
reticulum. Hydrocarbons are produced by decarboxylation
of the long chain acids via an intermediate aldehyde
(Buckner and Kolattukudy, 1973).

Diester waxes of 2 types, $RCO_2R'CO_2R''$ and $RCO_2R'O_2CR$,
are known (Nicolaides et al., 1970) and alkane diols of
the 1,2; 2,3 (Sawaya and Kolattukudy, 1973); α,ω (Tulloch,
1971; Tulloch and Hoffman, 1973) or $\alpha,\omega-1$ (Tulloch, 1970)
series have been characterized. Sawaya and Kolattukudy
(1972) found that the carboxyl carbon of a precursor acid
became the β-carbon (C-3) of the alkane-2,3-diols of the
uropygial gland. The components of the waxes from the
uropygial glands of swans (Bertelsen, 1974) and owls
(Jacob and Poltz, 1974) have recently been analyzed by gas
chromatography-mass spectroscopy. Fatty acids from the
swans suggested utilization of propionate units, 2,4,6-
trimethyl and 2,4,6,8-tetramethyl fatty acids, while those
from owl included 2-ethyl, 2-propyl, and 2-butyl branches.
The diester waxes of animal skin surfaces are also peculiar in the high proportion of branched chain structures
in the fatty acids and alkane-1,2-diols, 68% and 81%, respectively, in the dog, for instance (Nicolaides et al.,
1970). The jaw fat of the bottlenose dolphin (Ackman et

al., 1973b) and the head fat of the pilot whale (Blomberg, 1974) also contain branched wax esters with iso alcohols and acids, but are peculiar in having iso and anteiso pentanoic acids.

Production of fatty alcohols from fatty acids is a relatively straightforward two-step reduction known to occur in a number of tissues. Substrate specificity at this level affects the composition of wax esters and glyceryl alkyl ethers and alk-1-enyl ethers. Copepod wax esters contain fatty alcohols that are markedly less unsaturated than the fatty acids (Benson *et al.*, 1972).

XIII. Vitamin E

In the past, there has been considerable disagreement regarding the mode of action of vitamin E. The problem has been complicated by 1) multiple nutritional deficiency signs, 2) multiple forms of the vitamin, 3) replacement in whole or part by structurally unrelated synthetic lipid antioxidants, 4) dependence of the requirement on dietary levels of polyunsaturated fatty acids, PUFA, 5) biologically available selenium, 6) sulfur amino acids, and 7) the amelioration of the toxicity of various chemicals by therapeutic levels of the vitamin.

Vitamin E is believed to function largely, if not exclusively, as a lipid antioxidant *in vivo*, as outlined (Witting, 1975) in a highly simplified manner below.

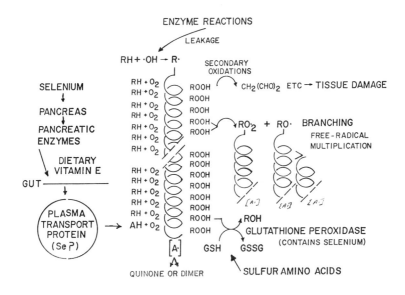

Fig. 2. A highly simplified outline of lipid peroxidation in vivo illustrating initiation, chain branching, termination, catabolism of primary products, and secondary reactions leading to tissue damage. See text for details. From Witting (1975). Reprinted by courtesy of the American Oil Chemists' Society.

Lipid peroxidation is initiated in part by free-radical leakage from enzymatic reactions. The normal metabolism of certain compounds is exceptionally "leaky." This is readily demonstrated *in vitro* as shown by Recknagel and Ghoshal (1966; Recknagel, 1967) with carbon tetrachloride and by DiLuzio with ethanol (DiLuzio and Costales, 1965; DiLuzio, 1966). The hepatic microsomal mixed-function oxidase system has been intensively studied because this system appears to be inherently exceptionally "leaky." Pfeifer *et al.* (1971; McCay *et al.*, 1972; Fong *et al.*, 1973) have presented data strongly suggesting that the leakage occurs during electron transport, probably at the flavin level, and involves the HO· free radical. Initiation of lipid peroxidation, $RH + HO· \rightarrow R· + H_2O$, occurs only during active metabolism (Johnson *et al.*, 1971; Morgan and DiLuzio, 1970) and has its origin in enzymatic reactions but is not a direct product of or bear a stoichiometric relation to such a reaction and should, therefore, be described as adventitious.

The primary product of lipid peroxidation is lipid bound fatty acid hydroperoxides, ROOH. These reactive molecules are "detoxified" by peroxidases, such as the selenium-containing enzyme glutathione peroxidase (Rotruck *et al.*, 1972; Rotruck *et al.*, 1973; Christopherson, 1968), $ROOH + 2GSH \rightarrow ROH + GSSG + H_2O$. The activity of this enzyme is affected by the dietary level of biologically available selenium (Chow and Tappel, 1974).

Vitamin E acts as a moderator between adventitious enzymatic initiation of lipid peroxidation and the enzymatic reduction of hydroperoxides to harmless compounds. The presence of such a moderator is necessary because free-radical initiated lipid peroxidation propagates via a cyclic chain reaction, capable of producing a large

$$R· + O_2 \rightarrow RO_2·$$
$$RO_2· + RH \rightarrow ROOH + R·$$

number of product molecules per individual initiation (Uri, 1961). Vitamin E, AH, withdraws free-radicals from the system and terminates the cyclic chain reaction by competing with lipid-bound fatty acids, RH, for reaction with the peroxy free-radicals, $RO_2·$, $RO_2· + AH \rightarrow ROOH + [A·]$ (Uri, 1961). The cyclic chain reaction can be competitively terminated by any fat-soluble lipid antioxidant that reaches the appropriate subcellular site (Witting,

1970).

Lipid hydroperoxides, aside from detracting from membrane stability, may react directly with proteins or may undergo secondary oxidation reactions resulting in scission of the fatty acid chain with the production of reactive aldehydes and dialdehydes. The cross-linking and polymerization of proteins by reaction of compounds, such as malondialdehyde, $CH_2(CHO)_2$, with the free amino groups of the basic amino acids is known to reduce or destroy enzymatic activity and to result in the formation of lipopigments of the ceroid and/or lipofuscin type (Chio and Tappel, 1969a; 1969b). This potential tissue damage is moderated by both vitamin E and selenium, but the 2 substances do not act in the same manner. Vitamin E does not prevent lipid peroxidation, but it does control or moderate the *yield* of hydroperoxide per adventitious free-radical initiation. A peroxidase, such as glutathione peroxidase, does not participate directly in lipid peroxidation, but does destroy the products of such reactions by reducing the lipid hydroperoxide group to a secondary alcohol group (Christopherson, 1968). Both agents, therefore, minimize the quantity of hydroperoxide available to produce tissue damage.

The actual balance of reactions in living tissues is much more complicated than has been indicated thus far, but these complications do not detract from the basic outline presented above.

Lipid peroxidation is an omnipresent, ongoing process, never completely under control as evidenced by the lifelong, progressive accumulation of age pigments of the lipofuscin and/or ceroid type (Strehler *et al.*, 1959). In Batten's disease, neuronal ceroid lipofuscinosis (Zeman and Dyken, 1969; Siakotos *et al.*, 1970), a genetic defect in a peroxidase (Armstrong *et al.*, 1974b) other than glutathione peroxidase, children with normal dietary and blood levels of vitamin E began to go blind at approximately 6 years of age and thereafter the brain atrophies and there is a massive accumulation of lipopigment amounting to as much as 5% of the *wet* weight of the brain. The adult form of the disease, Kuf's disease (Kornfeld, 1972) shows the same enzyme defect (Armstrong *et al.*, 1974a). Lipid peroxidation is not only not prevented by vitamin E, it is also not successfully minimized to a totally negligible level. The somewhat less massive accumulation of lipopigment in the liver and brain of chronic alcoholics will be discussed separately below.

It has been very difficult to separate the actions of vitamin E and selenium for several reasons which have only recently become apparent. Scott and co-workers (Thompson and Scott, 1970; Gries and Scott, 1972; Noguchi et al., 1973) have shown that selenium is required for maintenance of pancreatic function in the chick. Fibrosis of the pancreas in the selenium-deficient chick results in a vitamin E deficiency since the absorption of fat and this fat-soluble vitamin from the gut are severely impaired. Raising the dietary level of selenium from 0.005 ppm to 0.050 ppm increased the uptake of radioactive tocopherol from the gut to the bloodstream 100-fold (Thompson and Scott, 1970). There has also been some discussion of a vitamin E carrier protein which may also contain selenium (Desai et al., 1964).

Since vitamin E acts as a moderator between 2 enzymatic reactions, its action within the lipid membrane is to some extent equivalent to its action in a beaker of fat (Witting, 1965a; 1965b). Several general statements may be made regarding the moderating effect of vitamin E. The propagation rate, $RO_2{}^{\cdot} + RH \xrightarrow{k_p} ROOH + R^{\cdot}$, increases with the degree of unsaturation of the fatty acids (Uri, 1961) whereas the termination rate, $RO_2{}^{\cdot} + AH \underset{k_{-t}}{\overset{k_t}{\rightleftharpoons}}$ ROOH + [A$\cdot$], is not sensitive to fatty acid unsaturation (Uri, 1961). Vitamin E, RRR-α-tocopherol, is a relatively unhindered phenolic antioxidant whereas the antioxidants used to stabilize food (Chipault, 1962), petroleum (Nixon, 1962), and rubber (Bevilacqua, 1962) products are frequently hindered phenolics such as di- or tri-ter-butyl phenol. Such an unhindered phenolic antioxidant has an optimum concentration for the minimum rate of oxygen uptake and the ratio of $k_t : k_{-t}$ is relatively low (Mahoney, 1969; Mahoney, 1967).

As the PUFA content of the tissue lipids increase, as is currently happening in the American population (Witting and Lee, 1975), the yield of hydroperoxide per free-radical initiation increases. At the optimum concentration of vitamin E in oleate, linoleate, and linolenate *in vitro*, the yield of hydroperoxide is approximately 2-3, 70, and 140 molecules per initiation (Witting, 1969). Each initiation results in the "destruction" of a molecule of vitamin E at the termination of the cyclic chain reaction.

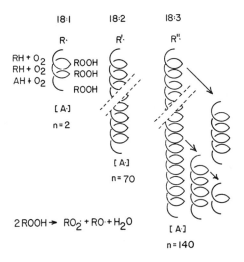

Fig. 3. The effect of the degree of fatty acid unsaturation on the yield of hydroperoxides prior to termination of the preradical initiated cyclic chain reaction by vitamin E. Chain branching results from the breakdown of products hydroperoxides with the initiation of new cyclic chain reactions. From Witting (1975). Reprinted by courtesy of the American Oil Chemists' Society.

Chain branching or free-radical multiplication occurs through secondary initiations originating from the breakdown of product peroxide, $ROOH \rightarrow RO^{\cdot} + {}^{\cdot}OH$ or $2ROOH \rightarrow RO_2^{\cdot} + RO^{\cdot} + H_2O$. Hydroperoxides from secondary initiations may also give rise to new free-radical initiations and so on *ad infinitum*. Since each primary initiation and each level of chain branching results in destruction of vitamin E, a basis for a variable vitamin E requirement related to the PUFA content of the tissue lipids exists (Witting,

1972a; 1972b; Witting, 1974). The phospholipid fatty
acids of a tissue such as skeletal muscle may, in response
to dietary lipids, vary in unsaturation from the *equivalent* of approximately pure linoleate to approximately pure
linolenate (Witting and Horwitt, 1964).

The system may become "uncontrolled" with the occurrence of tissue damage in several ways. Withdrawal of
dietary vitamin E and the depletion of tissue levels of
the antioxidant result in an increase in the yield of
hydroperoxide per primary adventitious free-radical initiation. This increases the potential for chain branching
or free-radical multiplication and the overloading of the
capacity to destroy hydroperoxides before they produce tissue damage. In matched groups of weanling rats being
depleted of vitamin E, the period required to produce
creatinuria as a sign of the onset of nutritional muscular
dystrophy varied from 3 weeks to 6 months depending on the
dietary supply of PUFA (Witting and Horwitt, 1964).

Selenium-deficiency results in a reduced capacity to
destroy hydroperoxides. Tissue damage may then occur at
relatively low levels of vitamin E-moderated hydroperoxide
production and there is also a greater potential concentration of hydroperoxides to give rise to free-radical
multiplication.

Temporarily or transiently increasing the level of
primary adventitious initiations through ingestion of
ethanol (DiLuzio and Costales, 1965; DiLuzio, 1966) or
carbon tetrachloride (Recknagel and Ghoshal, 1966;
Recknagel, 1967) or inhalation of ozone (Roehm *et al.*,
1972), the oxides of nitrogen (Thomas *et al.*, 1967), hy-
drazine derivatives (DiLuzio *et al.*, 1973) or hyperbaric
or pure oxygen (Johnson *et al.*, 1972; Kahn *et al.*, 1964)
has a somewhat different effect. The number of cyclic
chain reactions propagating simultaneously permits transient local buildups of hydroperoxide thus shifting the
equilibrium of the termination reaction, $RO_2\cdot + AH \rightleftharpoons ROOH + [A\cdot]$, toward the left. At this point, the hydroperoxide
yield per initiation rapidly increases by several orders
of magnitude despite the presence of residual antioxidant.
After the completion of, for instance, ethanol metabolism,
the rate of primary adventitious initiation returns to
"normal." Leftover hydroperoxides are enzymatically de-
stroyed and the residual vitamin E moderates hydroperoxide
production from "normal" adventitious initiations. Large

30

amounts of lipopigments accumulate in the brain and liver of the chronic alcoholic and, of course, gross tissue damage may eventually ensue.

Normal tissue vitamin E levels per gram of lipid correspond closely to the optimum concentrations required for the minimum rate of oxygen uptake *in vitro* (Witting, 1969; Witting, 1972a; 1972b; Witting, 1974). Under normal circumstances, increasing tissue levels of vitamin E detracts slightly from its efficiency as an antioxidant. Massively elevated tissue levels, which are difficult to produce and maintain, permit the organism to detoxify larger quantities of a hepatotoxin, such as ethanol, without incurring tissue damage or with less tissue damage than might otherwise occur. By increasing the tissue level of antioxidant, the transient concentration of hydroperoxide, [ROOH]/[AH], needed to essentially negate the termination reaction is also increased. The production of hydroperoxides proceeds at a moderated rather than an uncontrolled rate for a longer period.

When tissue damage has occurred under normal circumstances, the cyclic chain reaction must be unmoderated and the termination reaction negated. Administration of tracer doses of radioactive vitamin E and measurement of the relative rate of destruction (Green *et al.*, 1967; Bunyan *et al.*, 1967; Bunyan *et al.*, 1968; Diplock *et al.*, 1968; Green and Bunyan, 1969) yields no constructive information regarding the relative rate of lipid peroxidation. Under these circumstances, net vitamin E destruction is related to secondary reactions, such as quinone formation or dimerization of [A·].

The role of sulfur amino acids in this general scheme has not been clarified aside from glutathione production.

References

Ackman, R. G., and Hooper, S. N. (1973a). *Comp. Biochem. Physiol.* 46B, 153.

Ackman, R. G., Sipos, J. C., Eaton, C. A., Hilaman, B. L., and Litchfield, C. (1973b). *Lipids* 8, 661.

Adams, E. P., and Grey, G. M. (1970). *Chem. Phys. Lipids* 5, 198.

Albro, P. W., and Dittmer, J. C. (1970). *Lipids* 5, 320.

Anderson, R. G., Hussey, H., and Baddiley, J. (1972).
Biochem. J. 127, 11.

Anderson, W. H., Gellerman, J. L., and Schlenk, H. (1972).
Lipids 7, 710.

Armstrong, D. A., Dimmit, S., Boehme, D. H., Leonberg,
S. C., Jr., and Vogel, W. (1974a). *Science* 186, 155.

Armstrong, D., Dimmit, S., and Van Wormer, D. E. (1974b).
Arch. Neurol. 30, 144.

Bagby, M. O., Smith, C. R., Miwa, T. K., Lohmar, R. L.,
and Wolff, I. A. (1961). *J. Org. Chem.* 26, 1261.

Baker, N., and Lynen, F. (1971). *Eur. J. Biochem.* 19,
200.

Barnes, E. M., Jr., and Wakil, S. J. (1968). *J. Biol.
Chem.* 243, 2955.

Benson, A. A., Lee, R. F., and Nevezel, J. C. (1972). *In*
"Current Trends in the Biochemistry of Lipids" (J.
Ganguly and R. M. S. Smelie, eds.), p. 175. Academic
Press, New York.

Bergelson, L. D., Batrakov, S. G., and Pilipenko, T. V.
(1970). *Chem. Phys. Lipids* 4, 181.

Bertelsen, O. (1974). *Chemica Scripta* (preprint, p. 1).

Bevilacqua, E. M. (1962). *In* "Autoxidation and Antioxidants" (W. O. Lundberg, ed.), p. 857, v. 2. Interscience Publishers, New York.

Blank, M. L., Wykle, R. L., and Snyder, F. (1972).
Biochem. Biophys. Res. Commun. 47, 1203.

Bloch, K. (1969). *Accounts Chem. Res.* 2, 193.

Blomberg, J. (1974). *Lipids* 9, 461.

Blomquist, G. J., Soliday, C. L., Byers, B. A., Brakke,
J. W., and Jackson, L. L. (1972). *Lipids* 7, 356.

Bloomfield, D. K., and Bloch, K. (1960). *J. Biol. Chem.*
235, 337.

Bowen, D. M., Davidson, A. N., and Ramsey, R. B. (1974).
In "Biochemistry of Lipids," p. 141. University Park
Press, Baltimore.

Brett, D., Howling, H., Morris, L. J., and James, A. T.
(1971). *Arch. Biochem. Biophys.* 143, 535.

Buckner, J. S., and Kolattukudy, P. E. (1973). *Arch.
Biochem. Biophys.* 156, 34.

Bunyan, J., Green, J., Murrell, E. A., Diplock, A. T., and
Cawthorne, M. A. (1968). *Br. J. Nutr.* 22, 97.

Bunyan, J., Murrell, E. A., Green, J., and Diplock, A. T.
(1967). *Br. J. Nutr.* 21, 475.

Burger, M., and Glaser, L. (1966). *J. Biol. Chem.* 241,
494.

Burger, M. M., Glaser, L., and Burton, R. M. (1963). *J.
Biol. Chem.* 238, 2595.

Burton, R. M. (1974). *In* "Fundamentals of Lipid Chemistry" (R. M. Burton and F. C. Guerra, eds.), p. 373. BI-Science Publications, Missouri.

Butterworth, P. H. W., Burgos, J., and Hemming, F. W. (1966). *Arch. Biochem. Biophys.* 114, 398.

Castell, J. D., Lee, D. J., and Sinnhuber, R. O. (1972a). *J. Nutr.* 102, 93.

Castell, J. D., Sinnhuber, R. O., Lee, D. J., and Wales, J. H. (1972b). *J. Nutr.* 102, 87.

Chio, K. S., and Tappel, A. L. (1969a). *Biochem.* 8, 2821.

Chio, K. S., and Tappel, A. L. (1969b). *Biochem.* 8, 2827.

Chipault, J. R. (1962). *In* "Autoxidation and Antioxidants" (W. O. Lundberg, ed.), p. 478, v. 2. Interscience Publishers, New York.

Chow, C. K., and Tappel, A. L. (1974). *J. Nutr.* 104, 444.

Christopherson, B. O. (1968). *Biochim. Biophys. Acta* 164, 35.

Craig, B. M., and Bhatty, M. K. (1964). *J. Amer. Oil Chemists' Soc.* 41, 209.

Dart, R. K., and Kaneda, T. (1970). *Biochim. Biophys. Acta* 218, 189.

Davidoff, F., and Korn, E. D. (1962). *Biochem. Biophys. Res. Commun.* 9, 54.

Davidoff, F., and Korn, E. D. (1963). *J. Biol. Chem.* 238, 3199.

Desai, I. D., Calvert, C. C., and Scott, M. L. (1964). *Arch. Biochem. Biophys.* 108, 60.

Deuel, H. J., Jr. (1951). "The Lipids," v. 1. Interscience Publishers, Inc., New York.

DiLuzio, N. R. (1966). *Lab. Invest.* 15, 50.

DiLuzio, N. R., and Costales, F. (1965). *Exper. Mol. Pathol.* 4, 141.

DiLuzio, N. R., Stege, T. E., and Hoffman, E. O. (1973). *Exper. Mol. Pathol.* 19, 284.

Diplock, A. T., Cawthorne, M. A., Murrell, E. A., Green, J., and Bunyan, J. (1968). *Br. J. Nutr.* 22, 465.

Diringer, H., and Koch, M. A. (1973). *Z. Physiol. Chem.* 354, 1661.

Diringer, H., Marggraf, W. D., Koch, M. A., and Anderer, F. (1972). *Biochem. Biophys. Res. Commun.* 47, 1345.

Dunphy, P. S., Kerr, J. D., Pennock, J. F., and Whittle, K. J. (1966). *Chem. Ind.* 53, 1549.

Dunphy, P. J., Kerr, J. D., Pennock, J. F., Whittle, K. J., and Feeney, J. (1967). *Biochim. Biophys. Acta* 136, 136.

Earle, N. W., Slatter, B., and Burks, M. L., Jr. (1967). *J. Insect Physiol.* 13, 187.

Edwards, J. R., and Hayashi, J. A. (1965). *Arch. Biochem. Biophys.* 111, 415.

Elbein, A. D., Forsee, W. T., Schultz, J., and Laine, R. (1974). *J. Amer. Oil Chemists' Soc.* 51, 528A.

Erwin, J. A. (1973). *In* "Lipids and Biomembranes of Eukaryotic Microorganisms," p. 41. Academic Press, Inc., New York.

Erwin, J., and Bloch, K. (1964). *Science* 143, 1006.

Eto, T., Ichikawa, Y., Nishimura, K., Ando, S., and Yamakawa, T. (1968). *J. Biochem. (Tokyo)* 64, 205.

Feulgen, R., Imhauser, K., and Behrens, M. (1929). *Z. Physiol. Chem.* 180, 161.

Fong, K. L., McCay, P. B., Poyer, J. L., Keele, B. B., and Misra, H. (1973). *J. Biol. Chem.* 248, 7792.

Forsee, W. T., Laine, R. A., and Elbein, A. D. (1974). *Arch. Biochem. Biophys.* 161, 248.

Friedberg, S. J., and Heifetz, A. (1973). *Biochem.* 12, 1100.

Friedberg, S. J., Heifetz, A., and Greene, R. C. (1971). *J. Biol. Chem.* 246, 27.

Fulco, A. J. (1967). *Biochim. Biophys. Acta* 144, 701.

Fulco, A. J. (1969a). *J. Biol. Chem.* 244, 889.

Fulco, A. J. (1969b). *Biochim. Biophys. Acta* 187, 169.

Fulco, A. J. (1970). *J. Biol. Chem.* 245, 2985.

Fulco, A. J. (1974). *Ann. Rev. Biochem.* 43, 215.

Fulco, A. J., Levy, R., and Bloch, K. (1964). *J. Biol. Chem.* 239, 998.

Gellerman, J. L., and Schlenk, H. (1964). *Experentia* 20, 426.

Gellerman, J. L., and Schlenk, H. (1968). *Anal. Chem.* 13, 739.

Ginsburg, V. (1972). *Adv. Enzymol.* 36, 131.

Gough, D. P., Kirby, A. L., Richards, J. B., and Hemmings, F. W. (1970). *Biochem. J.* 118, 167.

Green, J., and Bunyan, J. (1969). *Nutr. Abs. Rev.* 39, 321.

Green, J., Diplock, A. T., Bunyan, J., McHale, D., and Muthy, L. R. (1967). *Br. J. Nutr.* 21, 69.

Greenspan, M. D., Birge, C. H., Powell, G. L., Hancock, W. S., and Vagelos, P. R. (1970). *Science* 170, 1203.

Gries, C. L., and Scott, M. L. (1972). *J. Nutr.* 102, 1287.

Groessman, A., and Scheren, H. (1855). *Ann. Chem.* 94, 230.

Gurr, M. I. (1974). *In* "Biochemistry of Lipids" (T. W. Goodwin, ed), p. 181. University Park Press, Baltimore.

Gurr, M. I., and James, A. T. (1971). "Lipid Biochemistry." Cornell University Press, New York.

Gurr, M. I., Robinson, M. P., and James, A. T. (1969). *Eur. J. Biochem.* 9, 70.

Gurr, M. I., Robinson, M. P., James, A. T., Morris, L. J., and Howling, D. (1972). *Biochim. Biophys. Acta* 280, 415.

Hajra, A. K. (1970). *Biochem. Biophys. Res. Commun.* 39, 1037.

Hakomori, S., Siddiqui, B., Li, Y. T., Li, S. C., and Hellerqvist, C. G. (1971). *J. Biol. Chem.* 246, 2271.

Hakomori, S., Stellner, K., and Watanabe, K. (1972). *Biochem. Biophys. Res. Commun.* 49, 1061.

Hancock, J. C., and Baddiley, J. (1972). *Biochem. J.* 127, 27.

Hancock, A. J., and Kates, M. (1973). *J. Lipid Res.* 14, 422.

Handa, S., Yamato, K., Ishizuka, I., Suzuki, A., and Yamakawa, T. (1974). *J. Biochem. (Japan)* 75, 77.

Harrington, G. W., Beach, D. H., Dunham, J. E., and Holz, G. G., Jr. (1970). *J. Protozool.* 17, 213.

Haskins, R. H. (1950). *Can. J. Res.* 28(C), 213.

Hemming, H. W. (1974). *In* "Biochemistry of Lipids" (T. W. Goodwin, ed.), p. 39. University Park Press, Baltimore.

Hilditch, T. P. (1940). "The Chemical Constitution of Natural Fats," p. 324. John Wiley and Sons, Inc., New York.

Hirschberg, C. B., and Kennedy, E. P. (1972). *Proc. Natl. Acad. Sci. USA* 69, 648.

Hopkins, C. Y., Chisholm, M. J., and Prince, L. (1966). *Lipids* 1, 118.

Ishibashi, T., Kijimoto, S., and Makita, A. (1974). *Biochim. Biophys. Acta* 337, 92.

Ito, S., Koyama, Y., and Toyama, Y. (1963). *Bull. Chem. Soc. Japan* 36, 1439.

Jacob, J., and Poltz, J. (1974). *J. Lipid Res.* 15, 243.

Jacobson, B. S., Kannangara, C. G., and Stumpf, P. K. (1973a). *Biochem. Biophys. Res. Commun.* 51, 487.

Jacobson, B. S., Kannangara, C. G., and Stumpf, P. K. (1973b). *Biochem. Biophys. Res. Commun.* 52, 1190.

James, A. T. (1972). *In* "Current Trends in the Biochemistry of Lipids" (J. Ganguly and R. M. S. Smelie, eds.), p. 49. Academic Press, Inc., New York.

Jamieson, G. R., and Reid, E. H. (1969). *Phytochem.* 8, 1489.

Jamieson, G. R., and Reid, E. H. (1972). *Phytochem.* 11, 1423.

Jarvis, F. G., and Johnson, M. J. (1949). *J. Amer. Oil Chemists' Soc.* 71, 4124.

Jefferts, E., Morales, R. W., and Litchfield, C. (1974). *Lipids* 9, 244.

Johnson, O., Hernell, O., Fix, G., and Olivecrona, T. (1971). *Life Sci.* 10(IL), 553.

Johnson, W. P., Jefferson, D., and Menzel, C. E. (1972). *Aerospace Med.* 43, 943.

Joseph, J. D. (1974). *J. Amer. Oil Chemists' Soc.* 51, 515A.

Kahn, H. E., Jr., Mengel, C. E., Smith, W., and Horton, B. (1964). *Aerospace Med.* 35, 840.

Kaneda, T. (1971). *Biochem. Biophys. Res. Commun.* 43, 298.

Kass, L. R., Brock, D. J. H., and Bloch, K. (1967). *J. Biol. Chem.* 242, 4418.

Kates, M., and Deroo, P. W. (1973). *J. Lipid Res.* 14, 438.

Kenyon, C. N. (1972a). *J. Bacteriol.* 109, 827.

Kenyon, C. N., Rippka, R., Stanier, R. Y. (1972b). *Arch. Mikrobiol.* 83, 216.

Kijimoto, S., Ishibashi, T., and Makita, A. (1974). *Biochem. Biophys. Res. Commun.* 56, 177.

Kleiman, R., Earle, F. R., Wolff, I. A., and Jones, Q. (1964). *J. Amer. Oil Chemists' Soc.* 41, 459.

Kleiman, R., Rawls, M. H., and Earle, F. R. (1972). *Lipids* 7, 494.

Klenk, E. (1965). *Adv. Lipid Res.* 3, 1.

Klenk, E., and Eberhagen, D. (1962). *Z. Physiol. Chem.* 328, 189.

Klenk, E., Knipprath, W., Eberhagen, D., and Koof, H. P. (1963). *Z. Physiol. Chem.* 334, 44.

Klenk, E., and Steinbach, H. (1959). *Z. Physiol. Chem.* 316, 31.

Knapp, A., Kornblatt, M. J., Schacter, H., and Murray, R. K. (1973). *Biochem. Biophys. Res. Commun.* 55, 179.

Kolattukudy, P. E., and Buckner, J. S. (1972a). *Biochem. Biophys. Res. Commun.* 46, 801.

Kolattukudy, P. E., Buckner, J. S., and Brown, L. (1972b). *Biochem. Biophys. Res. Commun.* 47, 1306.

Korn, E. D. (1964). *J. Lipid Res.* 5, 352.

Korn, E. D., Greenblatt, C. L., and Lees, A. M. (1965). *J. Lipid Res.* 6, 43.

Kornblatt, M. J., Schacter, H., and Murray, R. K. (1972). *Biochem. Biophys. Res. Commun.* 48, 1489.

Kornfeld, M. (1972). *J. Neuropath. Exper. Neurol.* 31, 668.

Kuhn, R., and Baer, H. H. (1956). *Chem. Ber.* 89, 504.

Kuhn, R., and Gauhe, A. (1962). *Chem. Ber.* 95, 518.

Lahav, M., Chiu, T. H., and Lennarz, W. J. (1969). *J. Biol. Chem.* 244, 5890.

Laine, R., Sweeley, C. C., Li, Y. T., Kisic, A., and Rapport, M. M. (1972). *J. Lipid Res.* 13, 519.

Lemieux, R. U. (1953). *Can. J. Chem.* 31, 396.

Lyman, R. L., Fosmire, M. A., Giotas, C., and Miljanich, P. (1970). *Lipids* 5, 583.

Lyman, R. L., Giotas, C., Fosmire, M. A., and Miljanich, P. (1969). *Can. J. Biochem.* 47, 11.

Lynen, F. (1972). *In* "Current Trends in the Biochemistry of Lipids" (J. Ganguly and R. M. S. Smelie, eds.), p. 5. Academic Press, New York.

Mahoney, L. R. (1967). *J. Amer. Oil Chemists' Soc.* 89, 1895.

Mahoney, L. R. (1969). *Angew. Chem.* 81, 555.

Martensson, E. (1963). *Acta Chem. Scand.* 17, 1174.

Martensson, E. (1966). *Biochim. Biophys. Acta* 116, 521.

McCay, P. B., Pfeifer, P. M., and Stipe, W. H. (1972). *Ann. N. Y. Acad. Sci.* 203, 62.

Miller, R. W., Earle, F. R., Wolff, I. A., and Barclay, A. S. (1968). *Lipids* 3, 43.

Morgan, J. C., and DiLuzio, N. R. (1970). *Proc. Soc. Exper. Biol. Med.* 134, 462.

Morice, I. M. (1967). *J. Sci. Food Agr.* 18, 343.

Nicolaides, N., Fu, H. C., and Ansari, M. N. A. (1970). *Lipids* 5, 299.

Nixon, A. C. (1962). *In* "Autoxidation and Antioxidants" (W. O. Lundberg, ed.), p. 695, v. 2. Interscience Publishers, New York.

Noguchi, T., Langevin, M., Combs, C. F., Jr., and Scott, M. L. (1973). *J. Nutr.* 103, 444.

Norton, W. T., and Brotz, M. (1963). *Biochem. Biophys. Res. Commun.* 12, 198.

Osborn, M. J. (1966). *Ann. N. Y. Acad. Sci.* 133, 375.

Oshino, N. (1972a). *Arch. Biochem. Biophys.* 149, 378.

Oshino, N., and Sato, R. (1972b). *Arch. Biochem. Biophys.* 149, 369.

Paltauf, F., and Holasek, A. (1973). *J. Biol. Chem.* 248, 1609.

Peleg, E., and Tietz, A. (1973). *Biochim. Biophys. Acta* 306, 168.

Pfeifer, P. M., and McCay, P. B. (1971). *J. Biol. Chem.* 246, 6401.

Pieringer, R. A. (1972). *Biochem. Biophys. Res. Commun.* 49, 502.

Pieringer, R. A., and Ganfield, M. W. (1974). *J. Amer. Oil Chemists' Soc.* 51, 528A.

Powell, R. G., Smith, C. R., Jr., and Wolff, I. A. (1967). *Lipids* 2, 172.

Pugh, E. L., and Kates, M. (1973). *Biochim. Biophys. Acta* 316, 305.

Radunz, A. (1967). *Phytochem.* 6, 399.

Raetz, C. R. H., and Kennedy, E. P. (1972). *J. Biol. Chem.* 247, 2008.

Ramsey, R. B., and Nicholas, H. J. (1972). *Adv. Lipid Res.* 10, 143.

Rao, K. S., and Pieringer, R. A. (1970). *J. Neurochem.* 17, 483.

Recknagel, R. O. (1967). *Pharmacol. Rev.* 19, 145.

Recknagel, R. O., and Ghoshal, A. K. (1966). *Lab. Invest.* 15, 132.

Reiser, R., Murty, N. L., and Rakoff, H. (1962). *J. Lipid Res.* 3, 56.

Roehm, J. N., Hadley, J. G., and Menzel, D. B. (1972). *Arch. Environ. Health* 24, 237.

Rotruck, J. T., Pope, A. L., Ganther, H. E., Swanson, A. B., Hafernan, D. G., and Hoekstra, W. G. (1973). *Science* 179, 588.

Rotruck, J. T., Pope, A. L., Ganther, H. E., and Hoekstra, W. G. (1972). *J. Nutr.* 102, 689.

Rowland, R. L., Latimer, P. H., and Giles, J. A. (1956). *J. Amer. Oil Chemists' Soc.* 78, 4680.

Sawaya, W. N., and Kolattukudy, P. E. (1972). *Biochem.* 11, 4398.

Sawaya, W. N., and Kolattukudy, P. E. (1973). *Arch. Biochem. Biophys.* 157, 309.

Scher, M., and Lennarz, W. J. (1969). *J. Biol. Chem.* 244, 2777.

Schlenk, H. (1970). *Prog. Chem. Fats Lipids* 9, 589.

Schlenk, H., and Gellerman, J. L. (1965). *J. Amer. Oil Chemists' Soc.* 42, 504.

Shaw, N. (1970). *Bact. Rev.* 34, 365.

Shaw, R. (1966). *Adv. Lipid Res.* 4, 107.

Siakotos, A. N., Watanabe, I., Saito, A., and Fleischer, S. (1970). *Biochem. Med.* 4, 361.

Siddiqui, B., and Hakomori, S. (1971). *J. Biol. Chem.* 246, 5766.

Siddiqui, B., Kawanami, J., Li, Y. T., and Hakomori, S. (1972). *J. Lipid Res.* 13, 657.

Siddiqui, B., and McCluer, R. H. (1968). *J. Lipid Res.* 9, 366.

Sinnhuber, R. O., Castell, J. D., and Lee, D. J. (1972). *Federation Proceedings* 31, 1436.

Smith, C. R., Jr., Bagby, M. O., Miwa, T. K., Lohmar, R. L., and Wolff, I. A. (1960). *J. Org. Chem.* 25, 1770.

Smith, C. R., Jr., Freidinger, R. M., Hagemann, J. W., Spencer, G. F., and Wolff, I. A. (1969). *Lipids* 4, 462.

Smith, C. R., Jr., Hagemann, J. W., and Wolff, I. A. (1964). *J. Amer. Oil Chemists' Soc.* 41, 290.

Smith, C. R., Jr., Kleiman, R., and Wolff, I. A. (1968). *Lipids* 3, 37.

Smith, P. F. (1970). *Biochim. Biophys. Acta* 280, 375.

Snyder, F. (1972). *Adv. Lipid Res.* 10, 233.

Snyder, F., Rainey, W. T., Jr., Blank, M. L., and Cristie, W. H. (1970). *J. Biol. Chem.* 245, 5853.

Spencer, G. F., Kleiman, R., Earle, F. R., and Wolff, I. A. (1969). *Lipids* 4, 99.

Spencer, G. F., Kleiman, R., Earle, F. R., and Wolff, I. A. (1970). *Lipids* 5, 277.

Spencer, G. F., Kleiman, R., Miller, R. W., and Earle, F. R. (1971). *Lipids* 6, 712.

Sprecher, H. (1968). *Lipids* 3, 14.

Sprecher, H. W. (1971). *Biochim. Biophys. Acta* 231, 122.

Sribney, M., and Kennedy, E. P. (1958). *J. Biol. Chem.* 233, 1315.

Stearns, E. M., Jr. (1970). *Prog. Chem. Fats Lipids* 9, 453.

Stone, K. J., Wellburn, A. R., Hemming, F. W., and Pennock, J. F. (1967). *Biochem. J.* 102, 325.

Strehler, B. L., Mark, D. D., Mildvan, A. S., and Gee, M. V. (1959). *J. Gerontol.* 14, 430.

Strominger, J. L., Higashi, Y., Sandermann, H., Stone, K. J., and Willoughby, E. (1972). *In* "The Biochemistry of the Glycosidic Linkage" (R. Piras and H. G. Pontis, eds.), p. 135. Academic Press, New York.

Stumpf, P. K., Vijay, I., and Harwood, J. L. (1972). *In* "Current Trends in the Biochemistry of Lipids" (J. Ganguly and R. M. S. Smelie, eds.), p. 57. Academic Press, New York.

Suzuki, K. (1972). *In* "Basic Neurochemistry" (R. W. Albers, G. J. Siegal, R. Katzman and B. W. Agranoff, eds.), p. 207. Little, Brown and Company, Boston.

Suzuki, A., Ishizuka, I., Ueta, N., and Yamakawa, T. (1973). *Jap. J. Exper. Med.* 43, 435.

Svennerholm, L. (1970). *In* "Lipid Metabolism" (M. Florkin and E. H. Stotz, eds.), p. 201. Elsevier Publishing Company, Amsterdam.

Svennerholm, L., Mansson, J. E., and Li, Y. T. (1973). *J. Biol. Chem.* 248, 740.

Takagi, T. (1964). *J. Amer. Oil Chemists' Soc.* 41, 516.

Taketomi, T., and Kawamura, N. (1972). *J. Biochem. (Tokyo)* 72, 799.

Talamo, B., Chang, N., and Bloch, K. (1973). *J. Biol. Chem.* 248, 2738.

Tayama, K., Schnoes, H. K., and Semmler, E. J. (1973). *Biochim. Biophys. Acta* 136, 212.

Thomas, H. V., Mueller, P. K., and Lyman, R. L. (1967). *Science* 159, 532.

Thompson, J. N., and Scott, M. L. (1970). *J. Nutr.* 100, 797.

Tornabene, T. G., and Markey, S. P. (1971). *Lipids* 6, 190.

Tsujimoto, M., and Toyama, Y. (1922). *Chem. Umschau, Fette, Ole, Wachse Harze* 29, 27.

Tulloch, A. P. (1970). *Lipids* 5, 247.

Tulloch, A. P. (1971). *Lipids* 6, 641.

Tulloch, A. P., and Hoffman, L. L. (1973). *Lipids* 8, 617.

Ullman, M. D., and Radin, N. S. (1973). *Trans. Amer. Soc. Neurochem.* 4, 95.

Ullman, M. D., and Radin, N. S. (1974). *J. Biol. Chem.* 249, 1506.

Uri, N. (1961). *In* "Autoxidation and Antioxidants" (W. O. Lundberg, ed.), p. 55, v. 1. Interscience Publishers, New York.

Uri, N. (1961). *In* "Autoxidation and Antioxidants" (W. O. Lundberg, ed.), p. 133, v. 1. Interscience Publishers, New York.

Vagelos, P. R. (1974). *In* "Biochemistry of Lipids" (T. W. Goodwin, ed.), p. 99. University Park Press, Baltimore.

Vance, W. R., Shook, C. P., III, and McKibbin, J. M. (1966). *Biochem.* 5, 435.

Van Der Horst, D. J. (1973). *Comp. Biochem. Physiol.* 46B, 551.

Volpe, J. J., and Vagelos, P. R. (1973). *Ann. Rev. Biochem.* 42, 21.

Wagner, H., and Konig, H. (1963). *Biochem. Z.* 339, 212.

Watkinson, R. J., Hussey, H., and Baddiley, J. (1971). *Nature* 229, 57.

Wellburn, A. R., and Hemming, F. W. (1966). *Nature* 212, 1364.

Wellburn, A. R., Stevenson, J., Hemming, F. W., and Morton, R. A. (1967). *Biochem. J.* 102, 313.

Wenger, D. A., Rao, K. S., and Pieringer, R. A. (1970). *J. Biol. Chem.* 245, 2513.

Wherrett, J. R. (1973). *Biochim. Biophys. Acta* 326, 63.

Wiegandt, H. (1971). *Adv. Lipid Res.* 9, 249.

Wiegandt, H. (1973). *Z. Physiol. Chem.* 354, 1049.

Wiegandt, H. (1974). *In* "Fundamentals of Lipid Chemistry" (R. M. Burton and F. C. Guerra, eds.), p. 347. BI-Science Publications, Missouri.

Wilkinson, S. G. (1969). *Biochim. Biophys. Acta* 187, 492.

Witting, L. A. (1965a). *Federation Proceedings* 24, 912.

Witting, L. A. (1965b). *J. Amer. Oil Chemists' Soc.* 42, 908.

Witting, L. A. (1969). *Arch. Biochem. Biophys.* 129, 142.

Witting, L. A. (1970). *Prog. Chem. Fats Lipids* 9, 519.

Witting, L. A. (1972a). *Amer. J. Clin. Nutr.* 25, 257.

Witting, L. A. (1972b). *Ann. N. Y. Acad. Sci.* 203, 192.

Witting, L. A. (1973). *Biochim. Biophys. Acta* 296, 271.

Witting, L. A. (1974). *Amer. J. Clin. Nutr.* 27, 952.

Witting, L. A. (1975). *J. Amer. Oil Chemists' Soc.* 52, 64.

Witting, L. A., and Horwitt, M. K. (1964). *J. Nutr.* 82, 19.

Witting, L. A., and Lee, L. (1975). *Amer. J. Clin. Nutr.* 28, 577.

Wykle, R. L., and Snyder, F. (1970). *J. Biol. Chem.* 245, 3047.

Zeman, W., and Dyken, P. (1969). *Pediatrics* 44, 570.

The Effect of Dietary Rapeseed Oil
on Cardiac Tissue

JOYCE L. BEARE-ROGERS

I.   Introduction

Dietary lipids have been primarily studied in relation
to hyperlipidemia and atherosclerosis, but here the concern
will rest with lipids that affect the myocardium. This
tissue appears to be particularly selective with respect to
substrates for fatty acid oxidation and may exhibit lipid
accumulation or cellular damage upon introduction of un-
suitable substrates.

Several reviews have already been written about the
effects of rapeseed oil on the heart (Rocquelin *et al.*,
1971; Aaes-Jorgensen, 1972; Abdellatif, 1972; Rocquelin *et
al.*, 1973a, 1973b; Mattson, 1973). In addition to rapeseed oil, brominated oils (Munro *et al.*, 1969, 1971), partially hydrogenated herring oil (Beare-Rogers *et al.*,
1972b), and a Polish substitute for cocoa butter (Ziemlanski and Krus, 1974) have also been associated with cardiac
necrosis and fibrosis.

Since rapeseed is well suited to northern climates,
its cultivation was encouraged in northern Europe and Canada. Rapeseed oil, also known as colza oil, has for the
last few years been Canada's major vegetable oil. Until
recently, erucic acid, *cis*-13-docosenoic acid, was the predominant fatty acid of this oil, but its content now does
not exceed 5% of the total fatty acids. This modification
in the fatty acid composition, achieved by selective plant
breeding, appeared to be nutritionally desirable as noted
below.

Roine (1960) and Rocquelin and Cluzan (1968) described
a condition designated as myocarditis in rats fed rapeseed
oil. Initially, these observations were difficult to rec-

43

oncile with the cardiac lipidosis in rats described by re-
searchers in the Netherlands (Thomasson et al., 1967; Abdellatif and Vles, 1970a). Subsequently it was established
that the nature of the lesions depended upon the duration
of the experiments.

II. Early Lipidosis

A. DETECTION AND DURATION

The accumulation of triglycerides as fatty droplets
in the myocardium occurs soon after feeding rats a source
of docosenoic acid. Ziemlanski et al. (1973) found that,
as soon as three hours after rats ingested a high erucic
rapeseed oil, lipidosis was evident in the heart. The most
extreme deposition of lipid in rats fed 60% of calories as
oil containing 48% erucic acid occurred between three and
six days after beginning the diet (Abdellatif and Vles,
1970a; Houtsmuller et al., 1970). In Fig. 1, the effects
of feeding Canadian rapeseed oil containing 33% erucic acid
to weanling rats for 4 weeks are seen. The level of the
oil was 20% by weight of the diet or 40% of calories. The
fatty acids in the heart reached peak accumulation in 1
week and thereafter decreased. The amount of erucic acid
present was also greatest at 1 week. With the control fat,
a 3:1 mixture of lard and corn oil, the cardiac fatty
acids at the time intervals studied remained relatively
low. Partially hydrogenated rapeseed oil containing 26%
C_{22} monoenoic acids and partially hydrogenated herring oil
containing 24% of these acids, but principally positional
isomers, also increased the deposition of lipids in the
heart, particularly at the early time intervals (Beare-
Rogers et al., 1971). Similar results on the early time
sequence of myocardial accumulation of lipid in rats fed
rapeseed oil have been obtained by Rocquelin et al. (1973b).

Many other groups of investigators have observed by
either chemical analysis or microscopy that fat accumulated
in the heart of rats fed high erucic rapeseed oil (Ziemlanski et al., 1972a, 1972b; Vodovar et al., 1972; Arrigo
and Ciangherotti, 1973; Dallachio et al., 1973; Jaillard
et al., 1973; Kramer et al., 1973). It is a condition that
is related to the amount of erucic acid in the diet and
that occurs in both sexes (Beare-Rogers et al., 1971;
Kramer, 1973). At a time when erucic acid appeared not to

be a readily available substrate, cardiac glycogen was utilized to a greater extent (Slinger *et al.*, 1973).

Lipidosis was not found in rats fed low erucic rapeseed oils (Beare-Rogers *et al.*, 1971; Rocquelin, 1972; Kramer *et al.*, 1973).

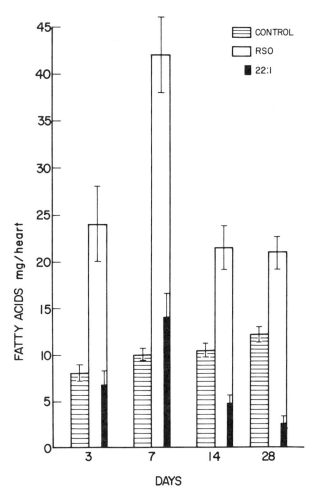

Fig. 1. Deposition of fatty acids in the heart of rats fed a control fat or rapeseed oil (RSO). Data from Beare-Rogers et al. *(1971).*

B. SYNTHESIZED OILS

Random triglycerides of tailored fatty acid composition, distinguished by a high level of either oleic acid, eicosenoic acid or erucic acid, were fed to weanling rats for 1 week to produce maximum lipid deposition (Beare-Rogers et al., 1972a). The dietary erucic acid produced pale fatty hearts and accounted for 36% of the total myocardial fatty acids. A low level of triglycerides was found with the high oleic oil, a somewhat higher level with eicosenoic acid oil, and a striking increase with the docosenoic acid (Beare-Rogers et al., 1972b). Dietary erucic acid also increased the level of cardiac free fatty acids, as observed by Rocquelin (1972). In all cases where there was an increase in cardiac lipids, all dietary fatty acids were represented in the cardiac deposits. Linoleic acid increased in both proportion and absolute amount, whereas the nondietary arachidonic acid decreased proportionately to other acids, but its absolute amount remained unchanged.

Abdellatif and Vles (1973a) who fed trierucate in an oil mixture found that cardiac lipidosis, assessed microscopically, was proportional to the docosenoic content of the diet. The evidence that erucic acid is a causative agent of lipid accumulation in the heart appears conclusive.

C. EFFECT OF AGE

The amount of cardiac fat deposited in one week was greater in young than in mature rats (Beare-Rogers and Nera, 1972). According to Abdellatif et al. (1974), the relative quantity of the accumulated fat at three days was similar in three and eleven week old rats, but the older rats exhibited a faster decrease. This, however, was offset by more myolysis and cell proliferation.

D. DIFFERENT SPECIES

Some of the most dramatic effects were observed in the duckling fed high erucic rapeseed oil (Abdellatif and Vles, 1970b, 1971, 1973b; Abdellatif et al., 1972). A severe hydropericardium, liver cirrhosis, and a high reticulocyte level occurred, in addition to lipid accumulation in the myocardium and skeletal muscles. The chick

46

exhibited myocardial fat deposits during the first two
weeks of rapeseed oil ingestion, but not after eight weeks
(Lall et al., 1972). Thereafter the chick resembled the
laying hen which was free from myocardial abnormalities
(Lall and Slinger, 1973). It must be remembered, however,
that attempts to find a well defined lymphatic system in
the chick have been unsuccessful. Since absorption is an
integral part of the nutritional process, any species lack-
ing a lymphatic system should not be seriously considered
for studies on lipids intended for extrapolation to mammals.

The rat, either of the Sprague-Dawley or Wistar
strain, has been the species most studied. The guinea pig,
hamster, and rabbit treated similarly also exhibited fatty
deposits in the myocardium (Abdellatif, 1972). There was
no evidence of elevated cholesterol levels or induced atherosclerosis in the rabbit fed 6% rapeseed oil (Kritchevsky et al., 1972). In the gerbil, the peak in lipid deposition was reached in four days when the total lipid accumulation was similar to that produced in the rat, but the
relative concentration of erucic acid was lower (Beare-
Rogers et al., 1972b). The commercial piglet fed skimmed
milk with the milk fat replaced by rapeseed oil appeared to
show less response than other animals tested, but microscopically its heart appeared to have more lipid droplets
(Beare-Rogers and Nera, 1972). The cardiac ultrastructure
of large pigs fed rapeseed oil indicated fat deposition
during the first twenty days, then regression, and the appearance of megamitochondria (Vodovar et al., 1973). A
few squirrel monkeys also showed some inability to metabo-
lize erucic acid (Beare-Rogers and Nera, 1972). Although
differences were observed in the extent and pattern of responses among the different animals, there appeared to be
no species which was free from an adverse effect to C_{22}
fatty acids.

E. RELATED FATTY ACIDS

A positional isomer of erucic acid, cetoleic acid
(cis,11-docosenoic acid), from herring oil caused in the
rat an accumulation of cardiac lipids approaching that of
erucic acid. An oil high in cis,11-eicosenoic acid produced a small amount of lipid deposition compared to that
of the docosenoic acids (Beare-Rogers et al., 1972a). The
extent of the effect was proportional to the C_{22} content
of the diet, as was demonstrated with partially hydrogen-

ated Canadian rapeseed and herring oils (Beare-Rogers *et al.*, 1972b) and with Norwegian capelin oil (Teige and Beare-Rogers, 1973). Supplying a relatively low level of long chain fatty acids from herring oil, Astorg and Rocquelin (1973) obtained negative results.

The C_{22} polyenoic acid of marine oil was shown to be converted during hydrogenation to a mixture of positional and geometric isomers (Lambertsen *et al.*, 1971). The long chain monoenoic isomers present in partially hydrogenated herring oil (Ackman *et al.*, 1971; Conacher *et al.*, 1972) were also deposited in cardiac tissue (Conacher *et al.*, 1973), as were the *cis* and *trans* monoenes of partially hydrogenated rapeseed oil (Quan and LeBreton, 1974).

In fully hydrogenated rapeseed oil, behenic acid was badly absorbed and did not affect the nature of cardiac lipids (Mattson and Streck, 1974).

F. COLD STRESS

Rats, six weeks of age rather than weanlings, were fed different diets at 4°C (Beare-Rogers and Nera, 1974). Although the period of acute lipid deposition in the heart lasted but a few days, it occurred during a period when the added stress of cold was critical. Rats fed a high erucic rapeseed oil had difficulty surviving the first week; those fed partially hydrogenated herring oil exhibited the same trend, particularly in the second week. Rats fed low erucic rapeseed oil resembled the control rats in withstanding the stress of cold. The timing of the high incidence of death in the cold coincided with the period of acute lipidosis in rats receiving C_{22} fatty acids.

G. MEMBRANE PHOSPHOLIPIDS

It has been well established that during lipid accumulation, much less erucic acid is incorporated into phospholipid than into triglycerides in the myocardium (Quan and LeBreton, 1972a, 1972b; Rocquelin *et al.*, 1973b; Bulhak-Jachymczyk *et al.*, 1974; Blomstrand and Svensson, 1974). These last investigators made the interesting observation that after 28 days the fatty acids of the mitochondrial cardiolipin contained somewhat more erucic acid than did those of other phospholipids. Cardiolipin, a constituent

of the inner mitochondrial membrane was found to be tightly bound to cytochrome oxidase (Awasthi *et al.*, 1971).

III.   Fate of Erucic Acid

A.   ABSORPTION AND TRANSPORT

Erucic acid has been shown to be readily absorbed
from the gastrointestinal tract (Deuel *et al.*, 1948, 1949;
Hornstra, 1972; Vaisey *et al.*, 1973). It appeared to be
even more available when it occurred in the 2-position of
triglycerides. Rocquelin (1973) demonstrated that interes-
terification of rapeseed oil augmented the cardiac lipidosis in the rat.

In a study of arterial-venous differences in concentration of fatty acids, Jaillard *et al.* (1973) demonstrated
that erucic acid was removed between the femoral artery
and the coronary sinus of man to an extent which was less
than that of oleic acid, but was similar to that of most
other fatty acids. Although erucic acid represented a relatively high proportion of the free fatty acids, it appeared not to be extracted by the rat heart in a preferential manner (Jaillard *et al.*, 1973). Rocquelin *et al.*
(1974) found no change in plasma lipid classes upon feeding rapeseed oil.

B.   ENTRANCE INTO MYOCARDIAL CELL

Fatty acid activation is surely not a problem in view
of the evidence to show that erucic acid enters the cardiac
cell. The fat droplets were found intracellularly (Vodovar
et al., 1972). However, Swarttouw (1974) found the specific activity of acyl CoA synthetase to be lower with erucic
than with palmitic acid. It is apparent that lipid accumulated within the cell when the erucic acid was not being
efficiently metabolized.

C.   MITOCHONDRIAL OXIDATION

The acyl CoA transfer across the inner mitochondrial
membrane involving carnitine acyltransferases has received
considerable attention. Erucyl carnitine inhibited the
oxidation of palmityl carnitine to a greater extent with

heart mitochondria than with liver mitochondria, but did not affect the formation of intramitochondrial long chain acyl CoA (Christophersen and Bremer, 1972a, 1972b). The amount of acyl-carnitines relative to the total carnitine in the heart appeared not be affected by the feeding of rapeseed oil (Gumpen and Norum, 1973). In each of the *in vitro* systems studied by Swarttouw (1974), the reaction with erucic acid was slower than that with palmitic acid.

The overall oxidation of radioactively labeled erucic acid, studied *in vitro* with cardiac mitochondria, was slower than that of palmitic or oleic acid (Lemarchal *et al.*, 1972; Swarttouw, 1974). By radioscanning myocardial lipids of rats given $14\text{-}^{14}\text{C}$-erucic or $10\text{-}^{14}\text{C}$-oleic acid, Ketevi *et al.* (1973) found a slower rate of metabolism for the C_{22} compound. This labeled erucic acid was converted to monoenoic fatty acids from C_{16} to C_{24}, whereas tritium-labeled oleic acid did not show corresponding conversions (Boucrot and Bezard, 1973).

The conclusion that erucic acid was transported into the mitochondria more slowly than palmitic or oleic acids probably does not pinpoint the rate-limiting step in erucic metabolism. The first step in β-oxidation involving acyl-dehydrogenase may be critical (Heijkenskjold and Ernster, 1974).

The oxidation of erucic acid by beating heart cells in culture involved chain-shortening to eicosenoic or oleic acid. It was clearly demonstrated that the carbon dioxide originating from the carboxyl group was produced well in advance of that from the fourteenth carbon of erucic acid (Pinson and Padieu, 1974).

The fetal heart appeared to be somewhat protected from the effects of long chain fatty acids. Using microscopic autoradiography after administering $14\text{-}^{14}\text{C}$-erucic acid or $10\text{-}^{14}\text{C}$-oleic acid to mice, Martinelli *et al.* (1973) found 100 times more radioactivity in the heart of the mother than in the 18 day old fetus.

ATP production, as assessed by ADP/O ratios, with different substrates was depressed in mitochondria from rats fed erucic acid (Houtsmuller *et al.*, 1970). This uncoupling of oxidative phosphorylation was not detected by Kramer *et al.* (1973).

D. CARDIAC AND HEPATIC ENZYMES

In rats fed rapeseed oil, either high or low in erucic acid, no alteration was apparent in the activities of myocardial lactate dehydrogenase, malate dehydrogenase, glucose-6-phosphate dehydrogenase, creatine phosphatase or ATPases (Dallacchio et al., 1973). Decreased adenyl cyclase activity in the heart of rats dosed with rapeseed oil was attributed to a decrease in catalytic sites (Cresteil et al., 1972). That the liver was involved in degrading erucic acid was suggested from observation of increased levels of nucleic acids, protein, and cytochrome P-450 in that organ (Gaillard et al., 1974). These investigators regarded erucic acid as a foreign compound which induced microsomal enzymes. On the other hand, Collomb et al. (1974) found no effects of erucic acid on hepatic endoplasmic reticulum.

E. REMOVAL OF CARDIAC LIPID

Coinciding with the period of acute cardiac lipidosis in rats fed high erucic rapeseed oil, the postheparin lipoprotein lipase of plasma increased (Struijk et al., 1973). Similarly, lipoprotein lipase activity in cardiac tissue was enhanced by rapeseed oil high in erucic acid (Jensen et al., 1974). The function of this enzyme in removing accumulated triglycerides could explain the later lipid regression.

IV. Necrosis and Fibrosis

A. OCCURRENCE

Some weeks or months after lipidosis has receded in the male rat, there is evidence of necrosis or fibrosis, probably preceded by myocytolysis. Unlike the even distribution for lipidosis, these lesions were much more evident in male than in female rats (Rocquelin and Cluzan, 1968; Kramer et al., 1973). The occurrence was shown to be dependent upon prolonged use of rapeseed oil, for when it was discontinued after one week, the fat deposits disappeared without causing long term lesions (Beare-Rogers and Nera, 1972).

The necrotic and fibrotic lesions have been well documented for the male rat, both from light microscopic stud-

ies and from electron microscopic studies (Abdellatif and
Vles, 1970a, 1971, 1973a; Vodovar *et al.*, 1972; Beare-Rogers *et al.*, 1972; Ziemlanski *et al.*, 1972a, 1972b). These
long term lesions were also reported for the pig (Vodovar
et al., 1973). There is a description of a similar condition in the heart of man attributed to an unknown cause
(Schlesinger, 1955).

It is appreciated that many conditions may cause cardiac necrosis or fibrosis, but the concern is with the factors that increase it above a background level in controlled studies. No group of workers looking for this
condition in male rats fed a high erucic oil failed to observe it. However, there is no unanimous agreement about
the properties of low erucic rapeseed oil (Abdellatif,
1972; Abdellatif and Vles, 1973a). It was first observed
by Rocquelin and Cluzan (1968) that a canbra oil, containing 1.9% erucic acid, was associated with the development
of long term lesions in the rat heart. Subsequently, this
observation with low erucic rapeseed oil was confirmed in
the same and other laboratories (Rocquelin *et al.*, 1973a;
Vodovar *et al.*, 1972; Kramer *et al.*, 1973; Beare-Rogers *et
al.*, 1974). Lesions were also found in the pig fed low
erucic oil (Levillain *et al.*, 1972).

That erucic acid *per se* was a cardiopathogenic agent
was convincingly demonstrated (Abdellatif, 1972; Abdellatif and Vles, 1973a). Similar conclusions were arrived
at by Beare-Rogers, Nera, and Craig (unpublished data)
from an experiment in which 30% erucic acid was interes-
terified with olive oil. This material caused a significant increase in cardiac lesions. The cause of lesions
with very low erucic rapeseed oils still needs an explanation.

After high erucic rapeseed oil has been fed to rats
for many months, there was but a low incorporation of erucic acid in cardiac lipids (Beare-Rogers *et al.*, 1972b;
Walker, 1972a; Kramer, 1973). Therefore, the morphological changes in the heart could hardly be associated with
its overall fatty acid composition.

B. PHOSPHOLIPIDS

Cardiac necrosis appears to follow disruption of cellular membranes. In view of this, the phospholipids were
studied in rats fed 20% rapeseed oil or olive oil for twen-

ty weeks (Beare-Rogers, unpublished data). Incorporation
of erucic acid had remained low, with less than 2% in the
fatty acids of phosphatidylcholine and phosphatidylethanolamine. The amount of total phospholipids did not differ
between the experimental groups. The most striking change
occurred in the distribution of the cardiac phospholipids
in which sphingomyelin increased three-fold in the rats
fed rapeseed oil (Table I).

The elevated concentration of cardiac sphingomyelin
was perhaps an indication of degenerative membranes coinciding with the occurrence of histologically observed necrosis.

Table I
DISTRIBUTION OF LIPID PHOSPHORUS IN CARDIAC PHOSPHOLIPIDS
OF RATS FED OLIVE OIL (OO) OR RAPESEED OIL (RSO)

Fraction[a]	P distribution %	
	OO	RSO
Card + PA	13.6 ± 0.3	13.0 ± 0.9[*]
PE	36.9 ± 1.0	31.1 ± 1.4[*]
PS + PI	4.2 ± 0.1	3.2 ± 0.5
PC	38.3 ± 1.4	36.2 ± 1.1[**]
Sphing	4.8 ± 0.7	13.5 ± 1.5[**]
Lyso PC	1.7 ± 0.9	2.6 ± 0.3

[a]Card, cardiolipin; PA, phosphatidic acid; PE, phosphatidylethanolamine; PS, phosphatidylserine; PI, phosphatidylinositol; Sphing, sphingomyelin; Lyso PC, lysophosphatidyl-
choline.
[*]Significantly different from the control group at the 5%
level of significance.
[**]Significantly different from the control group at the 1%
level of significance.

C. DIETARY MODIFICATIONS

A practical way of diminishing cardiopathogenic effect
of a dietary oil is dilution with other fats and oils. On
this basis, 10 cal % of a high erucic rapeseed oil (3 cal
% 22:1) appeared to be a no-effect level (Beare-Rogers *et
al.*, 1972b). Oro oil containing 2% or less of erucic acid
appeared not to differ from a control fat at 20 cal %, but
was significantly different at 40 cal % (Beare-Rogers *et
al.*, 1974). It was possible to dilute a high erucic rapeseed oil with other fats and oils to a level of erucic
acid close to that of low erucic oils and to achieve the
elimination of nutritional problems. A disturbing feature
of studies with low erucic oil was that there was still a
persistence of cardiac necrosis and fibrosis after sixteen
or more weeks.

Partial hydrogenation of Zephyr oil (less than 1%

erucic acid) eliminated its cardiopathogenic tendency
(Beare-Rogers *et al.*, 1974). Subsequently, a partial hydrogenation of Span Oil (Iodine Value 78) had the same effect (unpublished data). Approximately two-thirds of the
rapeseed oil used in Canada has been similarly treated.

The cause of concern with the *Brassica* oils was less-
ened by the conversion to low erucic seed and will hopeful-
ly diminish further once there is an understanding of the
nutritional improvement attained through partial hydrogenation of that oil. Admixture of low erucic rapeseed oil
with other vegetable oils has been nutritionally advanta-
geous, a situation which is justification for diversifica-
tion of oils in the food supply.

References

Aaes-Jorgensen, E. (1972). *In* "Rapeseed" (L. A. Appel-
    quist, and R. Ohlson), p. 301. Elsevier, New York.
Abdellatif, A. M. M. (1972). *Nutr. Rev.* 30, 2.
Abdellatif, A. M. M., Starrenburg, A., and Vles, R. O.
    (1972). *Nutr. Metab.* 14, 7.
Abdellatif, A. M. M., Timmer, W. G., and Vles, R. O.
    (1974). *J. Mol. Cell. Card.*, in press.
Abdellatif, A. M. M., and Vles, R. O. (1970a). *Nutr. Me-
    tab.* 12, 285.
Abdellatif, A. M. M., and Vles, R. O. (1970b). *Nutr. Me-
    tab.* 12, 296.
Abdellatif, A. M. M., and Vles, R. O. (1971). *Nutr. Me-
    tab.* 13, 65.
Abdellatif, A. M. M., and Vles, R. O. (1973a). *Nutr. Me-
    tab.* 15, 219.
Abdellatif, A. M. M., and Vles, R. O. (1973b). *Poul. Sci.*
    52, 1932.
Ackman, R. G., Hooper, S. N., and Hingley, J. (1971). *J.
    Amer. Oil Chem. Soc.* 48, 804.
Arrigo, L., and Ciangherotti, S. (1973). *Bull. Dell. Soc.
    Ital. Biol. Sper.* 49, 239.
Astorg, P., and Rocquelin, G. (1973). *C. R. Acad. Sci.*
    277, 797.
Awasthi, Y. C., Chuang, T. F., Keenan, T. W., and Carne,
    F. L. (1971). *Biochim. Biophys. Acta* 226, 42.
Beare-Rogers, J. L., and Nera, E. A. (1972). *Comp.
    Biochem. Physiol.* 41B, 793.
Beare-Rogers, J. L., and Nera, E. A. (1974). *Lipids* 9,
    365.

Beare-Rogers, J. L., Nera, E. A., and Craig, B. M. (1972a)
Lipids 7, 46.

Beare-Rogers, J. L., Nera, E. A., and Craig, B. M. (1972b).
Lipids 7, 548.

Beare-Rogers, J. L., Nera, E. A., and Heggtviet, H. A.
(1971). *Can. Inst. Food Tech. J.* 4, 120.

Beare-Rogers, J. L., Nera, E. A., and Heggtviet, H. A.
(1974). *Nutr. Metab.* 17, 213.

Blomstrand, R., and Svensson, L. (1974). *Lipids* 9, 771.

Boucrot, P., and Bezard, J. (1973). *Arch. Sci. Physiol.*
27, 1.

Bulhak-Jachymczyk, B., Kucharczyk, B. and Olszewska-Kaczyn-
ska, I. (1974). *Bull. de l'acad. polonaise des sci.*
22, 205.

Christophersen, B. O., and Bremer, J. (1972a). *FEBS
Letters* 23, 230.

Christophersen, B. O., and Bremer, J. (1972b). *Biochim.
Biophys. Acta* 280, 506.

Collomb, M. H., Albrecht, R., Griffaton, G., Manchon, P.,
and Lowy, R. (1974). *Enzyme* 18, 300.

Conacher, H. B. S., Page, B. D., and Beare-Rogers, J. L.
(1973). *Lipids* 8, 256.

Conacher, H. B. S., Page, B. D., and Chadha, R. K. (1972).
J. Amer. Oil Chem. Soc. 49, 520.

Cresteil, T., Ketevi, P., and Lapous, D. (1972). *C. R.
Acad. Sci.* 275, D, 1443.

Dallocchio, M., Larrue, J., Rabaud, M., Razaka, G.,
Crockett, R., and Bricaud, H. (1973). *C. R. Soc. Biol.*
167, 257.

Deuel, H. J., Jr., Cheng, A. L. S., and Morehouse, M. G.
(1948). *J. Nutr.* 35, 295.

Deuel, H. J., Jr., Johnson, R. M., Calbert, C. E., Gardner,
J., and Thomas, B. (1949). *J. Nutr.* 38, 361.

Gaillard, D., Pipy, B., and Derache, R. (1974). *Toxicol.*
2, 165.

Gumpen, S. A., and Norum, K. R. (1973). *Biochim. Biophys.
Acta* 316, 48.

Heijkenskjold, L., and Ernster, L. (1974). *Private Communication.*

Hornstra, G. (1972). *Nutr. Metab.* 14, 282.

Houtsmuller, U. M. T., Struijk, C. B., and Van der Beek, A.
(1970). *Biochim. Biophys. Acta* 218, 564.

Jaillard, J., Sezille, G., Dewailly, P., Fruchart, J. C.,
and Bertrand, M. (1973). *Nutr. Metab.* 15, 336.

Jansen, H., Hulsmann, W. C., Struijk, C. B., and Houtsmuller, U. M. T. (1974). *Biochim. Biophys. Acta*, in press.

Ketevi, P., Lapous, D., and Loriette, C. (1973). *J.
Physiol.* 67, 200A.

Kramer, J. K. G., Mahadevan, S., Hunt, J. R., Sauer, F. D., Corner, A. H., and Charlton, K. M. (1973). *J. Nutr.* 103, 1696.

Kritchevsky, D., Kim, H. K., and Tepper, S. A. (1972). *Atherosclerosis* 15, 101.

Lambertsen, G., Myklestad, H., and Braekkan, O. R. (1971). *J. Amer. Oil Chem. Soc.* 48, 389.

Lall, S. P., Pass, D., and Slinger, S. J. (1972). *Poul. Sci.* 51, 1828.

Lall, S. P., and Slinger, S. J. (1973). *Poul. Sci.* 52, 1729.

Lemarchal, P., Clouet, P., and Blond, J. P. (1972). *C. R. Acad. Sci.* 274, D, 1961.

Levillain, R., Vodovar, N., Flanzy, J., and Cluzan, R. (1972). *C. R. Soc. Biol.* 166, 1633.

Martinelli, M., Merlin, L., and Cohen, Y. (1973). *C. R. Acad. Sci.* 276, D, 853.

Mattson, F. H. (1973). "Toxicants Occurring Naturally in Foods," Second Edition, p. 189. National Academy of Sciences, Washington, D.C.

Mattson, F. H., and Streck, J. A. (1974). *J. Nutr.* 104, 483.

Munro, I. C., Middleton, E. J., and Grice, H. C. (1969). *Food Cosmet. Toxicol.* 7, 25.

Munro, I. C., Salem, F. A., Goodman, T., and Hasnain, S. H. (1971). *Toxicol. and App. Pharmacol.* 19, 62.

Pinson, A., and Padieu, P. (1974). *FEBS Letters* 39, 88.

Quan, P. C., and LeBreton, E. (1972a). *C. R. Acad. Sci.* 275, D, 1183.

Quan, P. C., and LeBreton, E. (1972b). *C. R. Acad. Sci.* 275, D, 1271.

Quan, P. C., and LeBreton, E. (1974). *C. R. Acad. Sci.* 278, D, 3123.

Rocquelin, G. (1972). *C. R. Acad. Sci. Paris* 274, 592.

Rocquelin, G. (1973). *Ann. Biol. Anim. Bioch. Biophys.* 13, 151.

Rocquelin, G., Astorg, P. O., Peleran, J. C., and Juaneda, P. (1974). *Nutr. Metab.* 16, 305.

Rocquelin, G., and Cluzan, R. (1968). *Ann. Biol. Anim. Biochim. Biophys.* 8, 395.

Rocquelin, G., Cluzan, R., Vodovar, N., and Levillain, R. (1973a). *Can. Nutr. Diet* 8, 103.

Rocquelin, G., Sergiel, J. P., Astorg, P. O., and Cluzan, R. (1973b). *Ann. Biol. Anim. Bioch. Biophys.* 13, 587.

Rocquelin, G., Sergiel, J. P., Martin, B., Leclerc, J., and Cluzan, R. (1971). *J. Amer. Oil Chem. Soc.* 48, 728.

Roine, P. E., Uksila, E., Teir, H., and Rapola, J. (1960). *Z. Ernahrungsw* 1, 118.

Schlesinger, M. J., and Reiner, L. (1955). *Amer. J. Path.* 31, 443.

Slinger, S. J., Coates B. J., Carney, J. A., and Walker, B. L. (1973). *Nutr. Rep. Int.* 8, 245.

Struijk, C. B., Houtsmuller, U. M. T., Jansen, H., and Hulsmann, W. C. (1973). *Biochim. Biophys. Acta* 296 253.

Swarttouw, M. A. (1974). *Biochim. Biophys. Acta* 337, 13.

Teige, B., and Beare-Rogers, J. L. (1973). *Lipids* 8, 584.

Thomasson, H. J., Gottenbos, J. J., Van Pijpen, P. L., and Vles, R. O. (1967). "Int. Symp. Chem. Technol. Rapeseed Oil and Other Cruciferae Oils," p. 381. Gdansk.

Vaisey, M., Latta, M., Bruce, V. M., and McDonald, B. E. (1973). *Can. Inst. Food Sci. Tech. J.* 6, 142.

Vodovar, N., Desnoyers, F., Cluzan, R., Marson, A. M., and Levillain, R. (1972). *C. R. Acad. Sci.* 274, D, 3109.

Vodovar, N., Desnoyers, F., Levillain, R., and Cluzan, R. (1973). *C. R. Acad. Sci.* 276, D, 1597.

Walker, B. L. (1972a). *Nutr. Metab.* 14, 8.

Walker, B. L. (1972b). *Can. J. Anim. Sci.* 52, 713.

Ziemlanski, S., Bulhak-Jachymczyk, B., Kucharczyk, B., Rusiecka, M., Opuszynska, T., Budzynska-Topolowska, J., Piekarzewska, A., Jakubowski, A., and Krasnodebski, P. (1972a). *Pol. Med. J.* 11, 1612.

Ziemlanski, S., Kucharczyk, B., and Bulhak-Jachymczyk, B. (1973). *Pol. Med. Sci. Hist. Bull.* 16, 563.

Ziemlanski, S., Opuszynska, T., and Krus, S. (1972b). *Med. J.* 11, 1625.

Ziemlanski, S., Opuszynska, T., Bulhak-Jachymczyk, B., Olszewska, I., Wozniak, E., Krus, S., and Szymanska, K. (1974). *Pol. Med. Sci. and Hist. Bull.* 15, 3.

Inborn Errors of Lipid Metabolism
and Lysosomal Storage Disorders

MICHEL PHILIPPART

I. Introduction

Excellent reviews are available on lysosomes (Dingle
and Fell, 1969; Dingle, 1973) and lysosomal disorders
(Stanbury et al., 1972; Hers and Van Hoof, 1973).

Lysosomes have elicited a great deal of interest since
they have been implicated in a growing number of human
diseases (Table I). Not unexpectedly, similar disorders
have been identified in other mammals (Table II) and presumably will be soon discovered in a variety of other living
organisms, since lysosomes are found not only in primitive
animals, but even in plants. This is an important development since, for ethical and practical reasons, human studies
are inherently piecemeal and limited to small numbers of
subjects. Man is likely to present with mutations causing
both more severe and milder abnormalities than would be detected in animals which have not escaped the imperatives of
natural selection and have shorter life spans. Many human
mutations, however, are likely to present genetic compounds
(McKusick et al., 1972). As attested by blood and histo-
compatibility groups, man has a great deal of genetic
heterogeneity in many proteins. Unless one deals with children issued from consanguineous unions or from inbred populations, many recessive disorders probably result from the
combinations of different mutations. This may explain the
growing number of atypical variants being reported. X-
linked disorders, however, offer an opportunity to study
single mutations in a given family. Even under these circumstances, variable expression is common (Johnston et al.,
1968) owing to the varying degree of inactivation of the
mutant gene from tissue to tissue or to multigenic interactions. Mutations affecting the rate of synthesis of a
product, for example, will be better and longer tolerated

59

Table I

Disease	Deficient enzyme	Natural substrate
Sphingolipidoses		
Farber	Ceramidase	Ceramide
Gaucher	β-glucosidase	Glucosyl ceramide
Krabbe	Cerebroside-β-galactosidase	Galactosyl ceramide
Sulfatidosis (metachromatic leukodystrophy)	Arylsulfatase A	Sulfatide Dihexosyl sulfatide
Sulfatidosis variant (multiple sulfatase deficiency)	Arylsulfatase A, B, and C Heparin sulfamidase Cholesterol sulfatase Dehydroepiandrosterone sulfatase	Sulfatide Dihexosyl sulfatide Mucopolysaccharides Cholesterol sulfate
Fabry	α-Galactosidase	Digalactosyl ceramide Trihexosyl ceramide Blood group substance B
Sandhoff	β-Hexosaminidase A and B	G_{M2}-ganglioside Globoside Oligosaccharide
Tay sachs	β-Hexosaminidase A	G_{M2}-ganglioside
Tay sachs AB variant	G_{M2}-ganglioside-β-hexosaminidase	G_{M2}-ganglioside
G_{M1}-gangliosidosis	β-Galactosidase	G_{M1}-ganglioside Oligosaccharide
Fucosidosis	α-Fucosidase	Antigen H Lewis blood substance Oligosaccharide
Niemann-Pick A and B	Sphingomyelinase	Sphingomyelin
Niemann-Pick "C" (A-variant Neutral lipid storage	Sphingomyelinase isozyme	Sphingomyelin
Wolman	Acid lipase	Triglyceride Cholesterol esters
Triglyceride storage	Acid lipase	Triglyceride
Cholesterol ester storage	Acid lipase	Cholesterol esters
Mucopolysaccharidoses		
Hurler	α-Iduronidase	Dermatan sulfate Heparan sulfate
Scheie	α-Iduronidase	Dermatan sulfate Heparan sulfate
Hunter	Iduronate sulfatase	Dermatan sulfate Heparan sulfate
Sanfilippo A	Heparin sulfamidase	Heparan sulfate
Sanfilippo B	α-Glucosaminidase	Heparan sulfate
Morquio	N acetylhexosamine 6-sulfate sulfatase	Chondroitin sulfate Keratin sulfate
Maroteaux-Lamy	Arylsulfatase B N acetylhexosamine 4-sulfate sulfatase	Dermatan sulfate
Mucopolysaccharidosis (variant)	β-Glucuronidase	Mucopolysaccharide
Carbohydrate storage		
Aspartylglucosaminuria	Aspartyl-glucosaminidase	Aspartyl-glucosamine
Mannosidosis	α-Mannosidase	Oligosaccharide
Pompe	α-Glucosidase	Glycogen
Phosphate storage ?	Acid phosphatase	?

by individuals also having an impairment of the catabolism of the same compound.

Touster (1973) has recently discussed some of the reasons for the dearth of solid chemical work on lysosomal

Table II
ANIMAL STORAGE DISORDERS

Disease	Animal	Reference
Gaucher	Dog	Jolly and Blakemore (1973)
Gaucher ?	Sheep	Laws and Saal (1968)
Gaucher ?	Pig	Sandison and Anderson (1970)
Krabbe	Terrier	Austin et al. (1968)
Krabbe	Miniature poodle	Zaki and Kay (1973)
G_{M2}-gangliosidosis	Pointer	Gambetti et al. (1970)
G_{M1}-gangliosidosis	Cat	Farrell et al. (1973)
G_{M1}-gangliosidosis	Calf	Donnelly et al. (1972)
Niemann-Pick	Cat	Chrisp et al. (1970)
Niemann-Pick	Mouse	Fredrickson et al. (1969)
Mannosidosis	Angus cattle	Hocking et al. (1972)
Glycogen storage	Dog	Mostafa (1970)

hydrolases. Complex logistics are involved in studying more than 40 enzymes (not including the isozymes) each being present in minute quantities and in variable proportions in different organs. Progress in the field depends, on the one hand, upon the improvement of basic analytical techniques and, on the other hand, upon the difficult integration between a number of highly specialized chemical, biochemical, and biological disciplines. I will focus here on more recent developments and problems deserving further investigation. I will also attempt to integrate some of the key information available.

II. Lysosomes and Cellular Turnover

A. LYSOSOMES AS A SPECIALIZED CELL COMPARTMENT

All biochemical reactions occurring in cells are precisely compartmentalized. Thus, genetic information is coded in the nucleus; macromolecules are synthesized in the endoplasmic reticulum, and energy is provided by the mitochondria. It is now becoming apparent that the degradation of macromolecules is also compartmentalized and probably takes place essentially, if not exclusively, *inside* the lysosomes. Cellular turnover has been recognized for

several decades, but the site of macromolecule degradation
has remained ill-defined.

The demonstration of the latency of the acid hydrolases in liver homogenates was the clue instrumental in
leading De Duve *et al.* (1955) to the discovery of lysosomes.
Somehow, from the procedural concept of latency emerged a
functional one, focusing on the danger that hydrolytic
enzymes represented for the cell containing them (De Duve
and Wattiaux, 1966). In that view, the main function of
the lysosomal membrane was to protect cell structures from
being digested. Much work was devoted to studying the factors capable of damaging or stabilizing the lysosomal membrane. Extracellular or intracellular release of lysosomal
enzymes was thought to be a damaging factor in some inflam-
matory disorders, such as arthritis (Weissmann, 1972). However, such hypotheses overlook the fact that the slightly
alkaline pH and buffer capacity of the cell sap and extracellular fluids would inactivate to a significant degree
the lysosomal hydrolases which all have an acid pH optimum.
The phenomenon of autophagy was later recognized as a mechanism of intracellular digestion compensating energy crises,
such as starvation. It took a long time to evolve the idea
that autophagy was but an exaggeration of a physiological,
discrete, continuous process.

B. INBORN LYSOSOMAL DISORDERS

Specific inherited deficiencies of a number of acid
hydrolases have now been characterized. Reflecting on one
of these deficiencies, Pompe disease, where glycogen storage occurs as a result of an α-glucosidase deficiency, Hers
(1965) formulated the concept of inborn lysosomal disorders.
Presently, we know 27 diseases which fall into that category. The main features of such disorders, as proposed by
Hers, are as follows: 1) presence of enlarged lysosomes
filled with undigestible material, 2) possible lack of
homogeneity of the material which may be cellular or extracellular in origin, 3) variation in intensity of storage
from one cell type to another, 4) progressivity, 5) variations in tolerance among different cell types, and 6) possibility of replacing the deficient enzyme, depending upon
the endocytic capacity of a given cell type.

Most, but, as we will discuss later, not all storage
diseases result from a specific deficiency in one of the

lysosomal acid hydrolases with the resulting accumulation of undegradable macromolecules inside the lysosomes. Could this represent a secondary mechanism used by a sick cell to put away certain types of accumulating substances? This does not seem to be the case, since in a disorder called I-Cell disease (mucolipidosis Type II and III), acid hydrolases are sharply decreased in skin fibroblasts, while macromolecules (phospholipids, glycolipids, mucopolysaccharides, etc.) accumulate together inside lysosomes (Philippart et al., 1973a). In other words, when one or several acid hydrolases are deficient, their corresponding substrates continue to be synthesized but cannot be properly degraded and start accumulating inside lysosomes. If the lysosomal function is more generally disturbed, all or most macromolecules also accumulate inside lysosomes. The accumulating substrate can be regarded as a biochemical *tracer* which indicates where these cell constituents normally end up. Thus, human pathology clearly indicates that lysosome function is essential for metabolic turnover.

C. VARIABILITY OF EXPRESSION

Striking differences between the clinical, pathological, and chemical features of these storage disorders have puzzled investigators. Indeed, many of these disorders involve the reticulo-endothelial system, as in Niemann-Pick disease, for example. Some of them involve mostly the nervous system, such as Tay-Sachs disease. Others spare it almost entirely, as illustrated in Fabry's disease.

Mucopolysaccharides may accumulate in fibroblasts from Fabry's disease, a classic "lipidosis" (Matalon et al., 1969). Oligosaccharides, presumably derived from partially degraded glycoproteins accumulate in the liver of patients with GM_1-gangliosidosis (Wolfe et al., 1974) or fucosidosis (Philippart, 1969). An abnormal oligosaccharide excretion has been reported in Sandhoff disease (Strecker and Montreuil, 1971). Gangliosides and glycolipids accumulate in mucopolysaccharidoses and in Niemann-Pick disease Type A and C (Philippart, 1972). The term "mucolipidosis" (Spranger and Wiedemann, 1970) has been proposed to accommodate overlapping between "lipidosis" and "mucopolysaccharidosis." This is still unduly restrictive and the expressions "lysosomal disease" or "lysosomal storage disorder" are certainly more apt.

How can we explain such a diversity if indeed we are witnessing basically identical processes? To answer this question, let us consider the factors involved in the cellular turnover. Lysosomal acid hydrolases are ubiquitous; they are found in most tissues and even extracellular fluids such as blood, lymph, urine, and cerebrospinal fluid. This ubiquitousness must have a great evolutionary advantage since it allows all cell types to degrade foreign materials to which they may be exposed through pinocytosis. Synthesis may be restricted to a few organs and even to one cell type. In other words, synthetic enzymes are the basis of what we call cellular differentiation. Thus, hemoglobin is synthesized exclusively by reticulocytes. Tyrosine can only be synthesized from phenylalanine by a specific liver enzyme, phenylalanine hydroxylase. Sulfatides are synthesized by a sulfotransferase found in the brain, kidney, and possibly gallbladder, but not in fibroblasts.

Since degradative enzymes are ubiquitous, genetic deficiencies can be detected in most tissues or body fluids, although some of these cells, being unable to synthesize the molecule involved in a given disease, need not have the corresponding degradative enzyme and therefore will not exhibit any disturbance as a result of a local enzyme deficiency. The reticulo-endothelial system represents a special case since these cells actively engage in phagocytosis and therefore are exposed to the ingestion of substances which they are unable to synthesize.

D. FIBROBLAST CULTURE

The use of tissue culture has allowed the investigation in a controlled environment of metabolic changes resulting from enzymatic deficiency. Skin fibroblasts, which are easy to obtain and grow, are now extensively used to diagnose or study metabolic disorders. It should always be kept in mind that culture conditions are artificial and subject to a number of pitfalls, such as infection by virus or mycoplasma, shift in pH, accelerated senescence, lack of hormonal controls, deficiency of oligoelements, and exposure to nutrients which might become toxic in certain conditions. In order to check this, it is important to determine not only biochemical parameters, such as enzyme activity or lipid distribution and concentration, but also morphological characteristics.

Electron microscopy (Kamensky *et al.*, 1973) is especially valuable in that respect, since it gives much more information than standard histological techniques. The ultrastructure of a piece of skin from which fibroblasts are grown furnishes a morphological base line which allows the distinction between culture artifacts and genuine pathology.

Normal cultured fibroblasts examined by electron microscopy contain mitochondria, endoplasmic reticulum, and a variety of inclusions. We will limit our discussion to the types of inclusions encountered, since the lysosomal disorders are generally manifested by the appearance of inclusion bodies. Cultured fibroblasts are prone to accumulate neutral lipids, mostly triglycerides. These appear as amorphous droplets which may merge with each other, reaching several microns in diameter. Labeled triglycerides are taken up by fibroblasts although very little is degraded or incorporated into phospholipids, even though triglyceride lipase is quite active in these cells (unpublished experiments). Lysosomes can be seen as dark granular bodies frequently in the vicinity of the Golgi apparatus where they are thought to be formed. They may be slightly dilated and appear then not as little bags, as has frequently been said, but as little sponges. Indeed, radiating from the limiting membrane, a delicate net of criss-crossing tracts can always be seen under proper conditions of cell fixation. Granular condensations may be observed in some of these spongy lysosomes. Residual bodies are few. They are considered to represent aged lysosomes which have accumulated digestive residues that cannot be further degraded. These residues appear as combinations of granular, lamellar, and amorphous material.

III. Primary Lysosomal Disorders

A. MUCOPOLYSACCHARIDOSES

Mucopolysaccharidoses represent a first group of lysosomal disorders characterized by the development of metachromatic inclusions. Upon electron microscopy (Kamensky *et al.*, 1973), these inclusions appear as spongy lysosomes which may become much larger than mitochondria. A number of small vacuoles can also be seen at the level of the hypertrophied Golgi apparatus. Some of the large vacuoles contain loose, thin lamellae, often in an onion bulb arrangement. We have observed a similar morphology in Hurler's, Hunter's, Scheie's diseases, and chondroitin-4-sulfate mucopolysaccharidosis. Metachromatic inclusions have been reported to occur in cultured fibroblasts not only in cases of mucopolysaccharidosis, but in about 30 different diseases including lipidoses as well as various genetic conditions which are obviously unrelated to storage disorders, such as myotonic dystrophy (Dorfman and Matalon, 1972). Following these observations, the diagnostic value of the metachromatic inclusions has been greatly reduced, but their biological significance should not be overlooked.

Such metachromatic inclusions can be easily obtained in normal cultures, being maintained at a nonphysiological alkaline pH (Lie *et al.*, 1972). The appearance of metachromasia seems linked to an accumulation of mucopolysaccharide in the lysosomal system. The increased concentration of mucopolysaccharide has been documented in cultured fibroblasts obtained from many disorders in which metachromatic inclusions have been found (Matalon and Dorfman, 1969). A significant difference, however, was observed in that the mucopolysaccharide distribution which was abnormal in the mucopolysaccharidoses, remained normal in the other conditions. Thus, mucopolysaccharide accumulation may result from the primary deficiency of a lysosomal hydrolase, from a physiological reaction to an excessively alkaline pH, or from unexplained reactions to a variety of genetic mutations.

Lysosomal enzymes all have an acidic optimal pH, and since lysosomes are thought to function physiologically at an acid pH (Jensen and Bainton, 1973), one can understand how excessive alkalinity may paralyze the digestive process. These interesting facts suggest a possible role for mucopolysaccharides in the lysosomal function (Hardin and Spicer, 1971). The increased synthesis of mucopolysaccharides occurring when the cells are placed in alkaline medium might represent the buffering mechanism involved in maintaining lysosomal acidity within the physiological range.

Lysosomal mucopolysaccharides might also affect enzyme activity and substrate dispersion. Mucopolysaccharides have been shown to form salts with proteins (Meyer *et al.*, 1937). They combine with lysosomal enzymes and alter their electrophoretic mobility (Kint *et al.*, 1973). In most mucopolysaccharidoses, many lysosomal activities are

greatly elevated, while β-galactosidase is generally decreased to about 25% of normal (Van Hoof and Hers, 1968).
Since these variations are found in genetically different
disorders, they obviously reflect a secondary phenomenon.
Part of the increased activity may simply result from the
increased number of lysosomes inside the storage cells.
But, however true, this explanation fails to take into
account the fact that several enzyme activities remain
within normal limits or are not significantly reduced (α-
fucosidase, β-glucosidase, and β-xylosidase), while other
activities beside β-galactosidase are decreased (α-galactosidase, sulfatase, and hyaluronidase) (Patel et al., 1970).
Basic enzymes can be inhibited by polyanions, such as
mucopolysaccharides. Electrostatic interaction depends on
the isoelectric point of the enzyme, the dissociation of
the carboxyl and sulfate groups and the salt concentration
(Mora and Young, 1958).

Mucopolysaccharides might also complex or trap water
insoluble substances, such as lipids. We do not know the
physiological way in which the enzymic hydrolysis of lipids
is accomplished. In the test tube, weak digestion may
occasionally be obtained in a micellar system, but a good
rate of degradation necessitates the introduction into the
system of natural (biliary salts) or artificial (Triton
X-100) detergents. Uncharacterized natural cofactors have
been shown to influence the degradation of sulfatide
(Jatzkewitz and Stinshoff, 1973), glucosyl ceramide (Ho and
O'Brien, 1971), and G_{M2}-ganglioside (Li et al., 1973). Deficiency in these cofactors might mimic lysosomal disorders
and are worth looking for.

It is unlikely that fibroblasts have available any
biliary salts for their lysosomal digestion. We have undertaken enzyme assays in which detergents are replaced by
chondroitin-4- and 6-sulfate or hyaluronic acid, to investigate how this affects sphingomyelinase activity. Preliminary results indicate that by using rather large concentrations of mucopolysaccharides, sphingomyelin hydrolysis
proceeds at a rate quite comparable to that obtained with a
detergent (Wolfe et al., 1974).

Lamellar formations observed in the tissues of patients with mucopolysaccharidosis most likely represent
lipids. Increased amounts of glycolipids have been demonstrated in these tissues (Philippart, 1972). This accumulation may result either from the inactivation of hydrolytic

enzymes or from an alteration of the natural dispersion factors. The increased glycolipid fraction may also be part of the lysosomal membrane which is proportionally increased in the storage cell (Huterer and Wherrett, 1974).

B. LIPIDOSES

Most of the work on acid hydrolases has been accomplished using artificial substrates. These enzymes have a limited specificity, only distinguishing the terminal moiety of the macromolecules on which they act. The mixed accumulation of cholesterol esters and triglycerides in acid lipase deficiency (Wolman's disease), or of G_{M1}-gangliosides and oligosaccharides in β-galactosidase deficiency, can be explained on that basis. Sphingomyelinase and cerebroside β-galactosidase activities, however, can only be determined against the natural substrates. The discovery of artificial substrates for these determinations would be most valuable. We have explored phosphodiesterase activity in Niemann-Pick disease A and C with this in mind. No correlation between phosphodiesterase and sphingomyelinase activity could be demonstrated, but abnormalities in one of the phosphodiesterase IV activities were detected (Callahan *et al.*, 1974a, 1974b). Ceramide lactosyl-β-galactosidase was implicated in a single case of lactosyl-ceramidosis, thought to represent a new type of sphingolipidosis (Dawson and Stein, 1970). The same activity, however, is also decreased in Krabbe's disease (Philippart *et al.*, 1974d; Wenger *et al.*, 1974). Great care is needed before making generalizations on these activities until a complete structural characterization of the lysosomal enzyme has been accomplished, as was done for lysozyme, for example (Chipman and Sharon, 1969).

Artificial substrates have also been useful for the demonstration of hydrolase isozymes. Some of these isozymes, such as the B isozyme of α-galactosidase (Beutler and Kuhl, 1972), have no demonstrated function as yet, and may account for the residual activity of the deficient enzyme often found in lysosomal diseases. Some isozymes possibly share a common subunit, although they act on different natural substrates. Conformational changes might also be involved (Tallman *et al.*, 1974). This may be the case for β-hexosaminidase; with both isozymes, A and B, being deficient in Sandhoff's disease (Sandhoff and Jatzkewitz, 1968) or arylsulfatase A, B, and C, all three being deficient in a variant of metachromatic leukodystrophy (Austin *et al.*, 1965).

Isoelectric focusing promises to be of help in studying isozymes of these enzymes which act upon natural substrates such as cerebroside-β-galactosidase (Suzuki and Suzuki, 1974), or sphingomyelinase (Callahan *et al.*, 1974).

In Gaucher's disease, a β-glucosidase deficiency results in storage of glucosyl ceramide. The bulk of the storage occurs in the spleen, or, when the patient has been splenectomized, in the liver and bone marrow. This rather localized storage seems related to membrane catabolism from red and white blood cells. Glucosyl ceramide being the basic unit from which the more complex neutral glycolipids or gangliosides which occur in all tissues are derived, it is surprising not to observe a widespread storage. Skin fibroblasts which actively synthesize trihexosyl ceramide would be expected to furnish lysosomes with a steady supply of undegradable glucosyl ceramide. However, ultrastructural examination of Gaucher fibroblasts fails to disclose the characteristic twisted crystalline structures observed in splenic histiocytes. Biochemically, there is only a discrete increase (2 to 4-fold) of glucosyl ceramide in these cultured fibroblasts. To explain this lack of frank storage, one may invoke three mechanisms. First, residual β-glucosidase activity in these fibroblasts may be sufficient to degrade the relatively small amount of substrate present. Second, glucosyl ceramide may serve as a precursor for resynthesis of the more complex glycolipids from which it derived. Third, fibroblasts may dispose of a mechanism to excrete glucosylceramide into the extracellular environment since it actually appears in the serum.

In metachromatic leukodystrophy, the absence of sulfatide inclusions in skin fibroblasts is easy to account for, since fibroblasts fail to synthesize detectable amounts of sulfatide. This can be demonstrated by studying incorporation of labeled acetate, galactose, or sulfate in these cells (Philippart, 1971a). No sulfatide is found under these conditions, despite the great sensitivity of the tracer techniques. Spongy dilated lysosomes, however, are observed in these cultures, but they are not as large as those found in the mucopolysaccharidoses (Kamensky *et al.*, 1973). Mucopolysaccharide concentration has not yet been determined in such cultures. The sulfatase deficiency may effect hypothetical sulfate esters which have escaped

detection so far. These in turn might interfere with the
normal lysosomal function, resulting in a compensatory
hypertrophy of the lysosomes without demonstrable functional deficiency or increase in hydrolase activity.

In Tay-Sachs disease, which results from a hexos-
aminidase A deficiency, the storage is even more closely
restricted to the brain than in metachromatic leukodystrophy. Tay-Sachs, or G_{M2}-ganglioside, is synthesized in the
brain only, although a trace amount of the substance has
occasionally been detected in the liver of these patients.
Skin fibroblasts do not exhibit abnormal inclusions upon
electron microscopy.

In a variant of Tay-Sachs disease known as Sandhoff
disease, both hexosaminidases A and B are deficient. Along
with G_{M2}-ganglioside storage in the brain, a tetrahexosyl
ceramide, called globoside, accumulates in the nonneural
organs. Skin fibroblasts contain a few onion bulb-like
inclusions objectivating the discrete storage of globoside
at their level. Interestingly, glycolipids isolated from
Sandhoff fibroblasts contain a slow moving ganglioside possibly related to G_{M2}-ganglioside, which is not detectable
in either control or Tay-Sachs fibroblasts. Since only
small quantities of this substance have been obtained, its
precise structure has not been determined, although it
probably will contain a terminal N-acetylgalactosamine or
N-acetylglucosamine moiety (Philippart *et al.*, 1974a).

G_{M3}-ganglioside accounts for 90% of fibroblast
gangliosides (Dawson *et al.*, 1973). Most of the remaining
lipid N-acetyl-neuraminic acid can generally be accounted
for by G_{D3}, the disialyl derivative of G_{M3}-ganglioside.
No structural work has been done to support claims for the
presence of G_{M2}-ganglioside in Tay-Sachs fibroblasts on the
basis of migration on thin-layer chromatography (Schneck
et al., 1973). Furthermore, the galactosaminyl transferase
which converts G_{M3} into G_{M2}-ganglioside, has been presented
as a neuronal marker being not demonstrable in a variety of
nonneural cell lines, including fibroblasts (Dawson *et al.*,
1973).

In Fabry's disease, an α-galactosidase deficiency
causes an accumulation of trihexosyl ceramide. This
glycolipid is synthesized by nonneural organs, including
skin fibroblasts, but apparently not by glial cells or
neurons (sympathetic and spinal ganglia representing an

exception to this rule) (Miyatake and Ariga, 1972). Dense
lamellated bodies with a regular periodicity can easily be
demonstrated in a skin biopsy as well as in fibroblasts
grown from it (Kamensky et al., 1973). The disease is sex-
linked, and as expected from the Lyon's hypothesis, females
have varying proportions of normal and deficient cells,
depending upon the random inactivation of the X-chromosome.
For unclear reasons, the proportion of inactivation of the
paternal compared to the maternal X-chromosome, can significantly differ from the 50-50% which is statistically expected. Some heterozygous females have a very low α-
galactosidase activity, and this may account for the symptoms they develop. Other females have an α-galactosidase
activity falling into the normal range. It is important
to be aware of the possibility of missing the detection of
a heterozygote on the basis of normal α-galactosidase
activity, normal glycolipid levels in blood and urine, and
absence of clinical symptoms such as corneal opacities
(Franceschetti et al., 1969; Philippart et al., 1969; Avila
et al., 1973). Therefore, it is advisable to biopsy the
skin of women at risk who seem to be biochemically normal,
and search for the characteristic inclusions in their skin
fibroblasts by electron microscopy (Philippart et al.,
1974b). Another way to study such females would be to clone
their fibroblasts in order to demonstrate the presence of
two cell populations, one having a deficient α-galactosidase activity (Romeo et al., 1970).

Niemann-Pick disease Type A is a lipid storage disorder, where sphingomyelin accumulates in most tissues following the deficiency of a specific lysosomal phosphodiesterase called sphingomyelinase. Electron microscopy of
cultured fibroblasts reveals a number of pleiomorphic inclusion bodies containing loosely arranged, onion bulb-like
lamellar material (Kamensky et al., 1973). Although an
absolute increase in sphingomyelin is observed in all nonneural organs, and to a lesser extent in the brains of
these patients, skin fibroblasts, despite the large number
of lipid-like inclusions at their level, do not contain an
excess of sphingomyelin. This does not appear to result
from a decreased rate of sphingomyelin synthesis in these
lines. The reason for this discrepancy is not known.

Niemann-Pick disease confronts us with a paradoxical
situation in which a profound sphingomyelinase deficiency
in Type A fibroblasts is not accompanied by a corresponding
sphingomyelin storage; while in Type C, sphingomyelin may

accumulate in the presence of a deficient sphingomyelinase isozyme (Callahan *et al.*, 1974) or even in the presence of an apparently normal complement of sphingomyelinase isozymes (unpublished observations).

IV. Secondary Lysosomal Disorders

There are many cases which pathologists are fond of calling lipidoses, or cases which clinicians would probably label mucolipidoses, in which lipid or mucopolysaccharide analysis and acid hydrolase determinations fail to reveal any definite abnormalities. Undoubtedly, many of the known lysosomal hydrolases have not yet been associated with a given clinical syndrome. At best, some increase in sphingomyelin concentration may suggest a diagnosis of Niemann-Pick disease Type C or sea-blue histiocytosis (Neville *et al.*, 1973). Minor abnormalities in neutral glycolipid or ganglioside distribution may be found. Upon electron microscopy, cultured fibroblasts are loaded with polymorphous lamellar or granular inclusions mixed with large spongy lysosomes similar to those described in Hurler's disease (Kamensky *et al.*, 1973). Histochemical reaction for acid phosphatase confirms the lysosomal nature of these inclusions. Instead of the characteristic increase in one or two related components in response to the specific deficiency in one of the lysosomal hydrolases, we are thus confronted by minor changes in the lipid composition of these cells.

The lysosomal membrane in the rat liver, compared to a liver homogenate or to mitochondria, is two-fold richer in sphingomyelin and twenty-fold richer in lysobisphosphatidic acid (Wherrett and Huterer, 1972), another phosphodiester recently detected in large concentration in Niemann-Pick tissues (Rouser *et al.*, 1968; Martin *et al.*, 1972). Lysosomal membranes are also enriched in glycolipids compared to the crude homogenate (Huterer and Wherrett, 1974). Cells accumulating inclusions might thus be considered as examples of "lysosomal membrane" storage reflected by a small increase in the sphingomyelin, lysobisphosphatidic acid and neutral glycolipids upon analysis of a total lipid extract. Under these circumstances, the distribution of the major lipids will remain normal. This brings us to envisage a different group of diseases in which all hydrolases may be normally active *in vitro* but not *in vivo*, as a result of some lysosomal dysfunction involving the lysosomal membrane, the lysosomal matrix, the lysosomal pH, or lysosomal cofactors.

Another type of secondary lysosomal storage disorder is constituted by the group of so-called amaurotic idiocies which comprises Jantzky-Bielschowsky, Spielmeyer-Vogt, and Kufs disease, also designated as Batten's disease, lipofuscinosis, or ceroid-lipofuscinosis. A specific peroxidase deficiency has been demonstrated in Kufs disease as well as in the prevalent form of Batten's disease, characterized by curvilinear bodies seen upon electron microscopy (Armstrong et al., 1974a). Genetic differences between these types have not yet been satisfactorily explained, but are known to exist in other conditions, such as G_{M1}-gangliosidosis or metachromatic leukodystrophy. A variety of peroxidases are known. With the exception of myeloperoxidase, which is apparently restricted to leukocytes, they are not present in lysosomes, but in some tissues, at least, they are associated with another cell organelle, the peroxisome (De Duve, 1969). Following the peroxidase deficiency in the ceroid-lipofuscinosis, peroxides accumulate (Armstrong et al., 1974b), damaging cell membranes, specifically, membrane lipids, polyunsaturated fatty acid being a choice target for peroxidation. Peroxidized lipids form complex pigment-like aggregates which probably cannot be digested by lysosomal hydrolases, owing to their compactness as well as to their insolubility. These aggregates, however, end up in the lysosomes as any other cell component following the physiological flux of the cellular turnover. Lipofuscin, the age pigment which accumulates during life, probably results from an essentially identical process involving localized, occasional deficiencies in the peroxidase system. We have demonstrated a generalized decrease in lipid turnover in a brain explant of a patient with lipofuscinosis (Philippart, 1971b). The lysosomal hydrolases studied in these patients have normal or only slightly increased activity, which suggests that these enzymes are resistant to or protected from peroxide damage. Lipids being soluble into other lipids, the pigment accumulating in the lysosomes may trap part of the membrane lipid entering the lysosome, protecting them from the action of the surrounding hydrolases.

In another disease described as sialuria (Fontaine et al., 1968), only one such patient who is still alive has been reported, N-acetylneuraminic acid is greatly elevated in plasma, urine, kidney, and liver. The condition might

be better designated as sialic or neuraminic acid storage
disease. A 3- or 4-fold increase of N-acetylneuraminic
acid is found in cultured fibroblasts. This increase is
not accompanied by much ultrastructural alteration. When
these cells were exposed to increasing amounts of N-acetylneuraminic acid in their growth medium, crystalline needles
appeared earlier in the cells from the patients with
sialuria than in the controls. N-acetylneuraminic acid may
either serve as a precursor to glycoprotein or ganglioside
which appears to be normally synthesized in these cells, or
it may be degraded by an aldolase into N-acetylmannosamine
and pyruvic acid. We have not been able to demonstrate the
existence of this aldolase in control fibroblasts (Philippart *et al.*, 1974c). To confirm that this is the enzyme
responsible for the disease, we will have to await the
availability of other tissues. N-acetylneuraminic aldolase
is probably not a lysosomal enzyme and thus, the disease
may represent another example of secondary lysosomal storage, where a product which would normally have been degraded before entering the lysosome, ends up there following the metabolic flux.

One way to investigate cellular capacity to deal with
an excess of a given substance is to feed it in large
quantity to cultured cells. In such circumstances, either
the hydrolytic capacity of the tested cells will be over-
whelmed and a situation comparable to a primary deficiency
can be expected, or the specific hydrolases will be sufficient and cell metabolism will not be significantly altered. In one experiment we conducted, cultured normal
fibroblasts did develop large inclusions when exposed to
excess sphingomyelin in their growth medium (5 mg/ml). The
ultrastructural appearance of these inclusions, however,
did not resemble that found in Niemann-Pick disease of
either Type A or C. Instead, worm-like inclusions were
observed. Somewhat similar inclusions have been seen in
Farber's disease, another lysosomal disorder due to a
ceramidase deficiency. Ceramides, being a product of the
action of sphingomyelinase on sphingomyelin, we thought
that the cells might be able to degrade the ingested
sphingomyelin, but that ceramidase, the enzyme involved in
the next degradation step, became rate-limiting, causing
secondary storage of ceramide. When analyzed, however,
ceramide levels in these fibroblasts were not significantly
increased while sphingomyelin accounted for 70% of the
phospholipids, and sphingomyelinase activity was much reduced. This illustrates the caution needed in evaluating

artificial models of storage disorders.

Yet another experimental method is to use poisons of
the lysosomal function. Two such agents have been used
for many years: chloroquine and retinol. Cultured fibroblasts exposed to microgram amounts of these substances
rapidly develop numerous polymorphous inclusions which are
large enough to become detectable by optical microscopy.
Chloroquine inclusions are rather similar to those observed
in Niemann-Pick and I-Cell diseases. Retinol, which may
selectively damage membranes, also gives rise to polymorphous inclusions. The notion that drugs may mimic lysosomal disorders at the ultrastructural level is an important one to keep in mind. Another drug, diethylamino-
ethoxyhexestrol, has been incriminated in an acquired lysosomal intoxication first considered to represent an adult
variety of Niemann-Pick disease (Yamamoto *et al.*, 1970).

Considering drug action illustrates how lysosomal
storage can result from a generalized impairment in lysosomal function.

A few years ago, studying fibroblasts from a variety
of patients with mucopolysaccharidosis, some of these
lines were found to be quite unusual in that they lacked
metachromasia and accumulated a striking number of inclusions having a refractile appearance when examined by phase
contrast microscopy (Leroy and Demars, 1967). These cells
were called I-(inclusion) cells and the disorder is known
as I-Cell disease or mucolipidosis II. Although they may
be clinically indistinguishable from Hurler's disease, urinary mucopolysaccharide excretion is normal, which gives an
important clue to the diagnosis. With the exception of
acid phosphatase and β-glucosidase, most hydrolases are severely deficient in fibroblasts and strikingly elevated in
the serum (Den Tandt *et al.*, 1974), urine, and cerebrospinal fluid (Wiesmann *et al.*, 1971a). Tissue and leukocyte
hydrolases tend to remain within normal limits, although β-
galactosidase may be depressed to 25% of the normal mean.
We have mentioned reduced activity of β-galactosidase as a
secondary nonspecific finding common to most mucopolysaccharidoses. In the brain or organs, there is little or no
apparent storage detectable by biochemical analysis or electron microscopy. I-Cell disease, then, is a multiple hydrolase deficiency essentially limited to fibroblasts and probably histiocytes. The greatly increased hydrolase activity
in body fluids, which has diagnostic value, has been ex-

plained as a leakage of lysosomal hydrolases from the fibroblasts (Wiesmann *et al.*, 1971b). The multiple hydrolase deficiency is accompanied by a failure in the degradation of lipids, mucopolysaccharides and to some extent, proteins. As a result, composite inclusions pile up in these cells. When studying incorporation of labeled precursors, the major fibroblast macromolecules seem normally synthesized though there is little turnover (Philippart *et al.*, 1973a). These fibroblasts behave as if they combined the mutations involved in the different lipidoses and mucopolysaccharidoses.

I-Cell disease is apparently not a primary lysosomal disorder. The leakage phenomenon may be compared with that observed in various intoxications with retinol (Weissman *et al.*, 1963), sucrose (Dingle *et al.*, 1969), nonmetabolizable sugars (Dingle, 1969) or chloroquine (unpublished experiments). Lysosomal enzymes from I-Cells are thought to have an abnormal carbohydrate moiety which prevents their recognition at the level of the fibroblast membrane (Hickman *et al.*, 1974). This brings to light a new aspect of lysosomal function. The existence of I-Cell disease points to an unsuspected differentiation which is peculiar to skin fibroblasts. It has been suggested that carbohydrates act as a chemical label which promotes the excretion of newly synthesized glycoprotein (Eylar, 1965) or more specifically determines the extracellular fate of protein molecules (Winterburn and Phelps, 1972).

V. Diagnosis

For screening purposes, enzyme assays have many advantages such as ease, low amount of material required, low cost, and rapidity.

Leukocytes (Kampine *et al.*, 1967) are useful but require time-consuming preparation. They represent a heterogeneous cell population, part of which has a low specific activity.

Urine is valuable when obtained fresh. Random specimens may not be representative and best results are obtained in aliquots of a 24 hour collection. Suitable specimens are often hard to obtain from young children or mentally retarded individuals. Some preparation is generally required, such as dialysis, concentration, or protein

precipitation. It remains the method of choice for diag-
nosing metachromatic leukodystrophy (arylsulfatase A deficiency). Many urinary acid hydrolases are not stable even
in the frozen state.

Serum or plasma may well become the preferred material,
since most assays require no more than 10 µl. Acidifica-
tion of the fresh specimen helps in stabilizing the activity for at least 48 hours (Den Tandt et al., 1974).

Most tissues can be used. Milligram amounts obtained
by needle biopsies from the liver or aspiration biopsies of
the intestine are perfectly suitable. Most tissue acid
hydrolases remain stable for years, but may become unstable following extraction. Tissues may also be kept lyoph-
ilized, which is a convenient and inexpensive way to mail
them.

Skin fibroblasts require tissue culture facilities,
but allow a practically unlimited number of determinations.
They can also be banked in liquid nitrogen for further
studies or shared with other investigators. Several months
are generally required to complete a comprehensive analysis.
The specific activity of hydrolases is much higher in fibroblasts than in leukocytes.

Lipid analysis is superior to enzyme determination in
the majority of cases where no precise clinical or pathological diagnosis is available. All cases labeled cerebral
palsy or mental retardation should be screened. Traditional
clinical criteria, such as onset in infancy or childhood,
progression or regression, organomegaly, increases the
likelihood of reaching a diagnosis, but will lead to ne-
glect of the significant number of atypical cases which are
now being discovered. The demonstration of cellular inclusions by the pathologist will always be a formal indication
for further biochemical investigation.

Lipid analysis has many advantages over enzyme analysis. Sphingolipids are remarkably stable and resistant
to denaturation. Total lipid extracts may be analyzed in
a matter of hours by qualitative or quantitative two-
dimensional thin-layer chromatography. The filter paper
technique (Philippart et al., 1969) is helpful for diag-
nosing metachromatic leukodystrophy (Philippart et al.,
1971), Fabry's disease (Philippart, 1972), Sandhoff
(Vidailhet et al., 1972), and Niemann-Pick disease Type A

(Philippart, 1974). Findings are less characteristic or
nonspecific in Gaucher's, Krabbe's, Niemann-Pick disease
Type C (Philippart, 1972), sea-blue histiocytosis, and
fucosidosis.

Five ml of serum allow a satisfactory glycolipid analysis. Characteristic abnormalities are found in Gaucher,
Fabry, and Sandhoff's diseases (Philippart, 1972; Vidailhet
et al., 1972).

A few mg of liver are sufficient for a complete phospholipid analysis. This will permit the diagnosis of the
different types of Niemann-Pick disease. Although large
amounts (about one gram of tissue) are needed for glycolipid analysis in the liver, small biopsy specimens are
sufficient to make the diagnosis of Gaucher's, Fabry's
disease, or fucosidosis.

Peripheral nerve may be the only tissue suitable to
confirm the increased galactosyl ceramide levels in
Krabbe's disease which in many ways differs from the typical lysosomal disease (Philippart, 1972; Philippart et al.,
1973b).

As a rule, a combination of lipid analysis and enzyme
determinations should be attempted. The demonstration of
an abnormal lipid distribution will indicate which enzyme
activities to determine. In case of conflicting data, more
refined techniques, such as pH curves or electrophoresis,
are mandatory.

The glycolipid and phospholipid analyses on cultured
fibroblasts have not been very helpful in our hands. Turnover studies after pulse labeling with ^{14}C-acetate and ^{14}C-
galactose reveal characteristic abnormalities in Farber's,
Fabry's, Sandhoff's, and I-Cell disease.

For heterozygote detection, skin fibroblasts are generally the material of choice, although leukocyte (Beutler
and Kuhl, 1970) or serum (O'Brien et al., 1972) may be
adequate in some diseases. The range of "normal" activity
almost always overlaps with the range of obligatory heterozygote activity. Some individuals will fall into that gray
zone and should be made aware of that uncertainty.

One should keep in mind the possible influence of
drugs, hormones, and toxic chemicals, the influence of

which has not been properly investigated. The wide normal range may be explained partly on the basis of the fact that our "normal" controls necessarily include various heterozygous deficiencies which may alter the enzyme distribution.

VI. Treatment of Lysosomal Disorders

A number of prerequisite conditions will have to be met before a successful treatment can be considered. These include early diagnosis and treatment (*in utero*, if ever possible). Key target organs should be reached. The activity should be supplied on a long-term, chronic basis without entailing toxic or immunologic reactions.

Correction of an inborn error of metabolism would require supplying either the normal gene or the normal enzyme itself.

A suitable amount of activity should be restored at least in the cells which bear the brunt of the disease, such as the central nervous system and the reticuloendothelial system. Since heterozygotes are most often symptom-free, half of the normal activity and possibly much less might be quite satisfactory. In many cases, cell damage occurs early during the fetal life, which would necessitate early diagnosis and treatment *in utero* unless we only succeed in increasing the survival of severely brain-damaged children.

Replacing the gene in a large cell population suggests techniques such as viral infection. Promising results have been obtained by this technique in fibroblasts deficient in galactose uridyl transferase, the enzyme deficient in galactosemia (Merril *et al.*, 1971). Possibly symbiotic, nonpathogenic bacteria or parasites might also be considered. The other alternative would be to supply the deficient enzyme itself. This approach is based upon the ability of cells to ingest foreign components by phagocytosis or pinocytosis (De Duve, 1964). This function, being highly developed in the reticuloendothelial system, the chance of success in those disorders where it is singly involved would be great. The central nervous system, on the other hand, is characterized by rather weak pinocytotic activity, and moreover, is effectively separated from the rest of the body by the blood-brain barrier and by the meninges which are highly intolerant to foreign substances (Austin, 1967).

Pinocytosis has been extensively studied in amoeba (Holter, 1959; Holter, 1965), and macrophages (Cohn and Parks, 1967). Although one has to be careful in extrapolating these data to human cells in general, it seems reasonable to assume that cells are capable of discriminating, to some extent, between substances present in the extracellular environment. Recent data indicates that specific sites on the fibroblast membrane are capable of recognizing a number of acid hydrolases, ensuring an efficient uptake (Hickman and Neufeld, 1972). Hydrolases prepared from placenta or urine are not taken up as efficiently as fibroblast hydrolases (Hickman *et al.*, 1974). It would be premature to conclude on that basis that one would have to administer a mixture of hydrolases from the organs to be treated in order to correct a given deficiency. Indeed, intravenously injected purified placental α-galactosidase was efficiently taken up by the liver of a man with Fabry's disease, where the recovered activity actually reached two- to four-fold the amount injected (Brady *et al.*, 1973). Pending more information about the intimate structure of hydrolases in various tissues, one may wonder whether fibroblast cultures represent a valid model for a study of replacement therapy. If one admits that hydrolases have to be excreted into the extracellular environment before being taken up, and then reaching the lysosomes, it becomes hard to understand why there is *pathological* evidence of two cell types in the heterozygote for Fabry's disease (Philippart *et al.*, 1974b). Indeed, the mutant cells are expected to share the α-galactosidase secreted by the normal cells. Although *in vivo*, islands of deficient cells might not have ready access to the functional enzyme, this situation would hardly prevail in monolayers bathed in a large quantity of culture medium.

A symposium has been devoted to the problems involved in replacement therapy (Bergsma, 1973). They are formidable and possibly insuperable for the time being. This should by no means discourage further exploration, especially if one starts taking advantage of the animal models now available.

The real breakthrough in the field has been prevention made possible through prenatal diagnosis and heterozygote detection. Prevention is a reality. One can reasonably expect that the speed, accuracy, and availability of screening methods will be further improved in the near future. The search for effective treatment is a challenging new frontier which will not be easily conquered.

Summary

Storage disorders involve the accumulation of a variety of macromolecules inside lysosomes. The existence of these diseases indicates that lysosomes have an important role in insuring the normal cellular turnover. As a rule, cellular damage will depend on the capacity of a given cell type to synthesize an undegradable compound in the presence of a generalized deficiency of an acid hydrolase. An isozyme deficiency may not be apparent when the total activity is measured with artificial or natural substrates, as illustrated by Tay-Sachs and Niemann-Pick disease Type C.

Mucopolysaccharides seem intimately involved in the lysosomal function. Little information is yet available on the mechanism regulating the proper dispersion of lipids or maintenance of an acid pH in the lysosomes.

Fibroblast culture, electron microscopy, and newly discovered animal models represent major tools available to unravel the lysosomal functions.

Aside from primary lysosomal storage disorders resulting from specific deficiencies in acid hydrolases, it is now becoming obvious that there is a heterogeneous group of lysosomal disorders secondary to toxic substances, substrate denaturation, deficiencies in natural cofactors or dispersing agents, abnormal membrane recognition sites, or mutations not involving the functional sites of the acid hydrolases.

Screening methods are being improved, but large-scale comprehensive screening is not yet practical. Prenatal diagnosis and heterozygote detection, although not always easy or failproof, represent major achievements in the prevention of these metabolic disorders. In a minority of selected cases, some form of enzyme replacement may be beneficial in checking the course of the disease.

ACKNOWLEDGMENTS

This work was supported in part by funds from the Mental Retardation Program, Neuropsychiatric Institute, UCLA, and Research Grants HD-04612, HD-00345, and HD-05615 from the National Institutes of Health.

Invaluable technical help was provided by Ms. Klaske Zeilstra, Mrs. Helen Roberson, Mr. Seiji Nakantani, and Elton Lassila.

References

Armstrong, D., Dimmit, S., and Van Wormer, D. E. (1974a). *Arch. Neurol.* 30, 144.

Armstrong, D., Van Wormer, D., Dimmit, S., Barber, D., and Neville, H. (1974b). *Trans. Amer. Soc. Neurochem.* 5, 135.

Austin, J., Armstrong, D., and Shearer, L. (1965). *Arch. Neurol.* 13, 593.

Austin, J. H. (1967). *In* "Inborn Disorders of Sphingolipid Metabolism" (S. M. Aronson and B. W. Volk, eds.), p. 359. Pergamon Press, Oxford.

Austin, J., Armstrong, D., and Margolis, G. (1968). *Trans. Amer. Neurol. Assoc.* 93, 181.

Avila, J. L., Conit, J., Velasquez-Avila, G. (1973). *Br. J. Dermatol.* 89, 149.

Bergsma, D. (1973). "Enzyme Therapy in Genetic Diseases," Birth Defects: Original Article Series, IX (2). Williams and Wilkins Company, Baltimore.

Beutler, E., and Kuhl, W. (1970). *J. Lab. Clin. Med.* 76, 747.

Beutler, E., and Kuhl, W. (1972). *Amer. J. Hum. Genet.* 24, 237.

Brady, R. O., Tallman, J. F., Johnson, W. G., Gal, A. E., Leahy, W. R., Quirk, J. M., and Dekaban, A. S. (1973). *N. Engl. J. Med.* 289, 9.

Callahan, J. W., Khalil, M., and Gerrie, J. (1974). *Biochem. Biophys. Res. Commun.* 58, 384.

Callahan, J. W., Lassila, E. L., and Philippart, M. (1974a). *Biochem. Med.* 11, 250.

Callahan, J. W., Lassila, E. L., and Philippart, M. (1974b). *Biochem. Med.* 11, 262.

Chipman, D. M., and Sharon, N. (1969). *Science* 165, 454.

Chrisp, C. E., Ringler, D. H., Abrams, G. D., Radin, N. S., and Brenkert, A. (1970). *J. Amer. Vet. Med. Assoc.* 156, 616.

Cohn, Z. A., and Parks, E. (1967). *J. Exp. Med.* 125, 213.

Dawson, G., and Stein, A. O. (1970). *Science* 170, 556.

Dawson, G., Stoolmiller, A. C., and Kemp, S. F. (1973). *Int. Soc. Neurochem.* 4, 298.

Den Tandt, W. R., Lassila, E. L., and Philippart, M. (1974). *J. Lab. Clin. Med.* 83, 403.

De Duve, C., Pressman, B. C., Gianetto, R., Wattiaux, R., and Applemans, F. (1955). *Biochem. J.* 60, 604.

De Duve, C. (1964). *Federation Proceedings* 23, 1045.

De Duve, C., and Wattiaux, R. (1966). *Ann. R. Physiol.* 28, 435.

De Duve, C. (1969). *Proc. R. Soc. Med. (B)* 173, 71.

Dingle, J. T., and Fell, H. B. (1969). "Lysosomes in Biology and Pathology" (J. T. Dingle and H. B. Fell, eds.). North-Holland Publishing Company, Amsterdam and London.

Dingle, J. T. (1973). "Lysosomes in Biology and Pathology." North-Holland Publishing Company, Amsterdam and London.

Dingle, J. T. (1969). *In* "Lysosomes in Biology and Pathology" (J. T. Dingle and H. B. Fell, eds.), p. 421. North-Holland Publishing Company, Amsterdam and London.

Dingle, J. T., Fell, H. B., and Glauert, A. W. (1969). *J. Cell Sci.* 4, 139.

Donnelly, W. J. C., Hannan, J., Sheahan, B. J., and O'Connor, P. J. (1972). *Vet. Rec.* 91, 225.

Dorfman, A., and Matalon, R. (1972). *In* "The Metabolic Basis of Inherited Disease" (J. B. Stanbury, J. B. Wyngaarden, D. S. Fredrickson, eds.), p. 1218. McGraw-Hill, New York.

Eylar, E. H. (1965). *J. Theor. Bio.* 10, 89.

Farrell, D. F., Baker, H. J., Herndon, R. M., Lindsey, J. R., and McKhann, G. M. (1973). *J. Neuropathol. Exp. Neurol.* 32, 1.

Fontaine, G., Biserte, G., Montreuil, J., Dupont, A., Farriaux, J. P., Strecker, G., Spik, G., Puvion-Dutilleul, F., Sezille, G., and Picque, M. T. (1968). *Helv. Paediatr. Acta* 23, 3.

Franceschetti, A. Th., Philippart, M., and Franceschetti, A. (1969). *Dermatologica* 138, 209.

Fredrickson, D. S., Sloan, H. R., and Hansen, C. T. (1969). *J. Lipid Res.* 10, 288.

Gambetti, L. A., Kelly, A. M., and Steinberg, S. A. (1970). *J. Neuropathol. Exp. Neurol.* 29, 137.

Hardin, J. H., and Spicer, S. S. (1971). *J. Cell Biol.* 48, 368.

Hers, H. G. (1965). *Gastroenterology* 48, 625.

Hers, H. G., and Van Hoof, F. (1973). "Lysosomes and Storage Diseases." Academic Press, Oxford.

Hickman, S., and Neufeld, E. F. (1972). *Biochem. Biophys. Res. Commun.* 49, 992.

Hickman, S., Shapiro, L. J., and Neufeld, E. F. (1974). *Biochem. Biophys. Res. Commun.* 57, 55.

Ho, M. W., and O'Brien, J. S. (1971). *Proc. Natl. Acad. Sci. USA* 68, 2810.

Hocking, J. D., Jolly, R. D., and Batt, R. D. (1972). *Biochem. J.* 128, 69.

Holter, H. (1959). *In* "International Review of Cytology" (G. H. Bourne and J. F. Danielli, eds.), p. 481, v. 8. Academic Press, New York and London.

Holter, H. (1965). *Symp. Soc. Gen. Microbiol.* 15, 89.

Huterer, S., and Wherrett, J. R. (1974). *Trans. Amer. Soc. Neurochem.* 5, 68.

Jatzkewitz, H., and Stinshoff, K. (1973). *FEBS Letters* 32, 129.

Jensen, M. S., and Bainton, D. F. (1973). *J. Cell Biol.* 56, 379.

Johnston, A. W., Weller, S. D. V., and Warland, B. J. (1967). *Arch. Dis. Child.* 43, 73.

Jolly, R. D., and Blakemore, W. F. (1973). *Vet. Rec.* 92, 391.

Kamensky, E., Philippart, M., Cancilla, P., and Frommes, S. P. (1973). *Am. J. Pathol.* 73, 59.

Kampine, J. P., Brady, R. O., and Kanfer, J. N. (1967). *Science* 155, 86.

Kint, J. A., Dacremont, G., Carton, D., Orye, E., and Hooft, C. (1973). *Science* 181, 352.

Laws, L., and Saal, J. R. (1968). *Aust. Vet. J.* 44, 416.

Leroy, J. C., and Demars, R. I. (1967). *Science* 157, 804.

Li, Y-T., Mazzotta, M. Y., Wan, Ch.-Ch., Orth, R., and Li, S.-Ch. (1973). *J. Biol. Chem.* 248, 7512.

Lie, S. O., McKusick, V. A., and Neufeld, E. H. (1972). *Proc. Natl. Acad. Sci. USA* 69, 2361.

McKusick, V. A., Howell, R. R., Hussels, I. E., Neufeld, E. F., and Stevenson, R. E. (1972). *Lancet* 1, 993.

Martin, J., Philippart, M., Van Hauwaert, J., Callahan, J., and Deberdt, R. (1972). *Arch. Neurol.* 27, 45.

Matalon, R., and Dorfman, A. (1969). *Lancet* 2, 838.

Matalon, R., Dorfman, A., Dawson, G., and Sweeley, C. C. (1969). *Science* 164, 1522.

Merril, C. R., Geier, M. R., and Petricciani, J. C. (1971). *Nature* 233, 398.

Meyer, K., Palmer, J. W., and Smyth, E. M. (1937). *J. Biol. Chem.* 119, 501.

Miyatake, T., and Ariga, T. (1972). *J. Neurochem.* 19, 1911.

Mora, P. T., and Young, B. G. (1959). *Arch. Biochem. Biophys.* 82, 6.

Mostafa, I. R. (1970). *Acta. Vet. Scand.* 11, 197.

Neville, B. G. R., Lake, B. D., Stephens, R., and Sanders, M. D. (1973). *Brain* 96, 97.

O'Brien, J. S., Okada, S., Chen, A., and Fillerup, D. L. (1972). *N. Engl. J. Med.* 283, 15.

Patel, V., Tappel, A. L., and O'Brien, J. S. (1970). *Biochem. Med.* 3, 447.

Philippart, M., Sarlieve, L., and Manacorda, A. (1969). *Pediatrics* 43, 201.

Philippart, M. (1969). *Int. Soc. Neurochem.* 2, 317.

Philippart, M. (1971a). *Soc. Pediatr. Res.* 81, 61.

Philippart, M. (1971b). *Int. Soc. Neurochem.* 3, 343.

Philippart, M., Sarlieve, L., Meurant, C., and Mechler, L. (1971). *J. Lipid Res.* 12, 434.

Philippart, M. (1972). *Adv. Exp. Med. Biol.* 25, 231.

Philippart, M., Nakatani, S., Kamensky, E., and Zeilstra, K. (1973a). *Pediatr. Res.* 7, 392.

Philippart, M., Nakatani, S., Zeilstra, K. (1973b). *Trans. Amer. Soc. Neurochem.* 4, 92.

Philippart, M. (1974). *N. Engl. J. Med.* 290, 284.

Philippart, M., Nakatani, S., Vidailhet, M., and Grignon, G. (1974a). *Pediatr. Res.* 8, 393.

Philippart, M., Kamensky, E., Cancilla, P., Sparkes, R. S., and Cotton, M. (1974b). *Pediatr. Res.* 8, 393.

Philippart, M., Kamensky, E., Cancilla, P., Callahan, J., Zeilstra, K., Nakatani, S., and Farriaux, J. P. (1974c). *Pediatr. Res.* 8, 393.

Philippart, M., Callahan, J. W., Klein, H., and Dichgans, J. (1974d). *Trans. Amer. Soc. Neurochem.* 5, 136.

Romeo, G., and Migeon, B. R. (1970). *Science* 170, 180.

Rouser, G., Kritchevsky, G., Yamamoto, A., Knudson, A., and Simon, G. (1968). *Lipids* 3, 287.

Sandhoff, K., Andreae, V., and Jatzkewitz, H. (1968). *Life Sci.* 7, 283.

Sandison, A. T., and Anderson, L. J. (1970). *J. Pathol.* 100, 207.

Schneck, L., Amsterdam, D., Brooks, St. E., Rosenthal, A. L., and Volk, Br. W. (1973). *Pediatrics* 52, 221.

Stanbury, J. B., Wyngaarden, J. B., and Fredrickson, D. S. (1972). "The Metabolic Basis of Inherited Disease" (J. B. Stanbury, J. B. Wyngaarden and D. S. Fredrickson, eds.). McGraw-Hill, New York.

Strecker, G., and Montreuil, J. (1971). *Clin. Chim. Acta* 33, 395.

Suzuki, Y., and Suzuki, K. (1974). *J. Biol. Chem.* 249, 2098.

Tallman, J. F., Brady, R. O., Quirk, J. M., Villalea, M., and Gal, A. E. (1974). *J. Biol. Chem.* 249, 3489.

Touster, O. (1973). *Mol. Cell Biochem.* 2, 169.

Van Hoof, F., and Hers, H. G. (1968). *Eur. J. Biochem.* 7, 34.

Vidailhet, M., Neimann, N., Grignon, G., Hartemann, P., Philippart, M., Paysant, P., Nabet, P., and Floquet, J. (1973). *Arch. Fr. Pediatr.* 30, 45.

Weissman, G. (1972). *N. Engl. J. Med.* 286, 141.

Weissman, G., Uhr, J. W., and Thomas, L. (1963). *Proc. Soc. Exp. Biol. Med.* 112, 284.

Wenger, D. A., Sattler, M., and Hiatt, W. (1974). *Proc. Natl. Acad. Sci. USA* 71, 854.

Wherrett, J. R., and Huterer, S. (1972). *J. Biol. Chem.* 247, 4114.

Wiesmann, U. N., Vassella, F., and Herschkowitz, N. N. (1971a). *N. Engl. J. Med.* 284, 1090.

Wiesmann, U. N., Lightbody, J., Vassella, F., and Herschkowitz, N. N. (1971b). *N. Engl. J. Med.* 284, 109.

Winterburn, P. J., and Phelps, C. F. (1972). *Nature* 236, 147.

Wolfe, L. S., Senior, R. G., and Ng-Ying-Kin, N. M. (1974). *J. Biol. Chem.* 249, 1828.

Wolfe, R., Philippart, M., Lassila, E., and Nakatani, S. (1974). *Pediatr. Res.* 8, 361.

Yamamoto, A., Adachi, S., Ishibe, T., Shinji, Y., Kakiuchi, Y., Seki, K., and Kitani, T. (1970). *Lipids* 5, 566.

Zaki, F. A., and Kay, W. J. (1973). *J. Amer. Vet. Med. Assoc.* 163, 248.

Intervention in Sphingolipid
Metabolism with Synthetic Inhibitors

NORMAN S. RADIN, KENNETH R. WARREN, RAMESH C. ARORA,
JUNG C. HYUN, AND RADHEY S. MISRA

For the past few years, this laboratory has been engaged in the synthesis of compounds which resemble in
structure the ceramides and cerebrosides. The basic structures are shown in Table I. The cerebrosides possess two

Table I

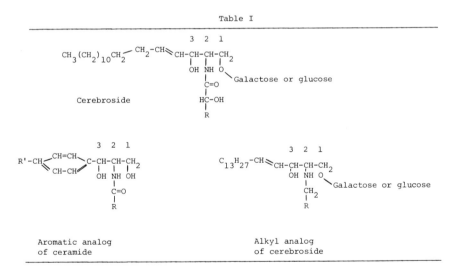

hydrolyzable linkages, the beta-glucoside link between
ceramide and a sugar, and the amide link between the long
chain base and the fatty acid. The formula shows sphingosine as the long chain base and the *trans* double bond is
drawn at an angle to emphasize the true shape. (This mode
of drawing also emphasizes the resemblance in shape to the
aromatic analog drawn at the lower left, since the benzene
ring has a similar bend.)

The first three carbon atoms of sphingosine are numbered in the table. Carbon 2 possesses the D configuration,
corresponding to D-amino acids (if C-1 were a carboxyl).
Carbon 3 also has the D configuration, which is generally
called the erythro form; the L configuration is the threo
form, which we have for some of the aromatic analogs. Many
galactocerebroside molecules also possess a hydroxyl group
on the fatty acid in the 2 position; this is also the D form,
but our synthetic compounds all have the DL form.

The lower two formulas illustrate two of our synthetic
approaches. The left-hand structure shows the replacement
of the long sphingosine side chain by a benzene ring, which
sometimes possessed a substituent in the para position. The
fatty acid moiety has been varied, in chain length and in
substituents, such as a hydroxyl group at the 2 position.
Some compounds have been made in which the fatty acid is replaced by a straight chain alkyl group, so that the nitrogen
atom is now a secondary amine, not an amide. The structure
on the right shows the latter approach, since the only change
in the cerebroside structure is replacement of the fatty acid
by an alkyl chain. At body pH, the secondary amines possess
a plus charge and are relatively soluble in water.

Before attempting to evaluate the compounds, we examined the conditions required for measuring the activity of
enzyme preparations enriched in galactocerebrosidase and
glucocerebrosidase. These enzymes act to hydrolyze the
glycosidic link shown in the upper formula. Ceramide and
free sugar are the products, neither of which has apprecia-
ble effect on the velocity of reaction. In the case of the
galactosidase, we have generally used a preparation from rat
brain (Bowen and Radin, 1969) which as been freed of much
protein and lipid. In the case of the glucosidase, we have
generally used a rat spleen homogenate or a partially purified enzyme from human placenta (Hyun *et al.*, 1975). It
should be noted that the two enzymes are distinct from a
number of other galactosidases and glucosidases, although
the specificity of the enzymes is still unclear.

The assay conditions for galactosidase are shown in
Table II (Radin and Arora, 1971). The substrate, galactocerebroside labeled in the galactose moiety, is emulsified
with a mixture of four different emulsifying agents, forming
a clear liquid. The enzyme is mixed with the substrate emulsion and citrate buffer pH 4.5. The oleate serves a specific
albeit unclear function, that is, it stimulates the enzyme

Table II

Galactocerebrosidase assay

Substrate
  1 mg stearoyl psychosine + 10 mg tween + 5 mg myrj + 3 mg
  tris oleate + 20 mg Na taurocholate + 5 ml water.
Medium
  1 ml containing enzyme + 0.1 mmole citrate (pH 4.5) + 137
  nmoles cerebroside (tritium-labeled). Incubate 3 hr at 37°.
Work-up
  Add 0.5 ml castor oil + isopropanol + chloroform + water,
  then vortex, count upper layer.

Inhibitors are added to incubation tube as dry film before other
components.

activity about 100%. The bile salt is very stimulatory,
and the nonionic detergents also have additive effects on
the observed activity. Unfortunately, the large amount of
detergent in the system makes partitioning a slightly risky
thing, since trace emulsions tend to form when methanol-
chloroform is added. We solved that problem by breaking
the emulsion, after incubation, with a solution of isopropanol, chloroform, and castor oil. The triglyceride is
added in large quantity to "soak up" the detergents and
keep them from producing emulsions. Under these conditions,
the radioactive galactose formed by the enzyme partitions
quite well into the water layer and can be counted.

The assay conditions for glucosidase are similar, as
shown in Table III. A phosphate-citrate buffer containing

Table III

Glucocerebrosidase assay

Substrate
  2 mg stearoyl psychosine + 10 mg tween + 5 mg myrj + 150
  mg Na taurocholate + 5 ml water.
Medium
  0.25 ml containing enzyme + 0.025 mmole citrate-phosphate-K^+
  (pH 5.4) + 55 nmoles cerebroside (C^{14} labeled).
Work-up
  Incubate at 37° for 30 minutes, extract ceramide with hexane
  from methanol-boric acid, backwash the hexane, count upper
  layer.

Inhibitors added as dried film before other components.

potassium ions proved to be better than a sodium citrate
buffer. In this case, we used glucocerebroside labeled with
[14C] stearic acid, which is easier to make than glucose-
labeled material. However, the partitioning system had to

be modified to allow us to count the ceramide portion instead of the sugar portion. It proved to be possible to separate cerebroside and ceramide quite well with a mixture of hexene-methanol-boric acid. The boric acid helps keep the cerebroside out of the hexane, presumably by forming a borate complex.

Data obtained with rat spleen glucosidase and a series of N-alkyl derivatives of glucosyl sphingosine (like the compound shown in the lower right side of Table I) is shown in Table IV. It is clear that all of these secondary

Table IV
INHIBITION OF RAT SPLEEN GLUCOSIDASE
BY N-ALKYL GLUCOSYL SPHINGOSINES
(INHIBITOR CONCENTRATION = 6 µM)

Alkyl chain	% Inhibition
Propyl	21
Butyl	42
Hexyl	85
Octyl	79
Decyl	74
Octadecyl	56

From Erickson and Radin (1973).

amines are potent inhibitors and that the best one is the N-hexyl compound. There is a rapid fall-off in effectiveness with shorter chains. This sort of sensitivity to alkyl or acyl chain length has been seen in many of our inhibitors.

A kinetic study made with rat spleen particles and two concentrations of hexyl psychosine (Erickson and Radin, 1973) clearly pointed to a competitive mode of inhibition, with a calculated K_i of 3×10^{-7} M. This is a very impressive inhibition constant. It is significant that the amine is very effective with glucocerebrosidase from mouse, rat, and human tissues, which suggests that the enzymes from these creatures are very similar. Moreover, the inhibitor is very effective when glucosidase activity is measured with nitrophenyl glucoside. Since there is much evidence that this kind of assay measures more than cerebrosidase activity, it means that the other glucosidase(s) is also inhibited and must have an active site that strongly resembles the active site in cerebrosidase.

A more detailed search for other inhibitors of glucosidase was made by preparing a large series of aromatic analogs of ceramide, as indicated in Table I. These were evaluated with a somewhat purified preparation of the enzyme from human placenta (Hyun *et al.*, 1975). A comparison of several amines with different chiral structures and substituents on the benzene ring is shown in Table V. All of them have an

Table V
DERIVATIVES OF 3-PHENYL-2-DECYLAMINO-1,3-PROPEDIOL TESTED
AGAINST PLACENTAL GLUCOCEREBROSIDASE (AT 0.3 mM)

Aromatic substituent	Configuration of carbons 2 and 3	Inhibition (% of control)
-	DL-erythro	98
-	L-threo	59
-	D-threo	39
P-nitro	DL-erythro	98
P-nitro	L-threo	52
P-nitro	D-threo	60
P-amino	DL-erythro	98
P-decanoylamido	DL-erythro	99

n-decyl side chain attached to the nitrogen atom. The first three lines show that the DL-erythro isomer was the best of the three isomers tested. Unfortunately, we did not have enough material to resolve the DL form; presumably the D form, which corresponds to the natural form of sphingosine, is more active than the mixture. The next three lines show the same relationship, but with a nitro group on the end of the molecule.

At the concentration tested (0.3 mM), the most active amines could not be compared in efficacy so a test was made at lower concentrations as shown in Table VI. The amines bearing a Para substituent were better than the unsubstituted benzene derivative. To our surprise, the compound most closely resembling ceramide--the one with the decanoyl group attached to the Para position--was no more active than the other two. However, it might be the most stable *in vivo*. The data given on the bottom lines show that a galactose group greatly weakened the effectiveness of the hexyl amine, but the glucosyl derivative was seen to be the best inhibitor of all. It is not surprising that the glucose moiety imparts additional binding power to the lipoidal amine, and it would be of great interest to test the glucosyl derivative of the aromatic compounds. The synthesis of such

91

Table VI
PLACENTAL GLUCOCEREBROSIDASE AND BRAIN GALACTOCEREBROSIDASE:
INHIBITION BY SECONDARY AMINES

Amine tested	Glucosidase			Galactosidase
	30 µM	6 µM	1.2 µM	6 µM
DPAPD[*]	82	28	2	7
P-nitro-DPAPD	92	66	19	5
P-amino-DPAPD	96	50	21	2
P-decanoylamido-DPAPD	91	68	23	5
N-hexyl-O-glucosyl- sphingosine	99	92	70	5
N-hexyl-O-galactosyl- sphingosine	21	5	1	3

[*]DPAPD = N-decyl-DL-erythro-3-phenyl-2-amino-1,3-propanediol. The numbers refer to %
inhibition at the different inhibitor concentrations.

compounds should be relatively straightforward.

The data in the third column shows that the best inhibitors are still potent even at 1.2 µM. On the other hand,
they are all rather inert toward galactocerebrosidase tested
in rat brain.

One of the best inhibitors in the aromatic series was
examined kinetically, with the expectation that it too (like
hexyl psychosine) would turn out to be a competitive inhibitor. A Hofstee plot, which is generally more reliable than
a Lineweaver-Burk plot, showed that the compound actually
acted as a mixed-type inhibitor, that is, part of it bound
to the catalytic site but most of it bound to some other
site and exerted an inhibitory action there too.

Additional examples of noncompetitive inhibition were
observed. A steroidal glucoside, deoxycorticosterone β-
glucoside, proved to be a modestly effective noncompetitive
inhibitor with K_i = 0.6 mM. This compound has been proposed
to be a naturally occurring component of mammals, but no
doubt its concentration is too low to interfere with glucocerebrosidase. p-Nitrophenyl glucoside, often used as a
substrate for assaying glucosidase, acted as a mixed-type
inhibitor. This observation probably means that it binds
to the catalytic site as a substrate and to the secondary
allosteric site as an inhibitor.

Phlorizin, a naturally occurring phenolic β-glucoside that interferes with glucose reabsorption by kidney was also tested. Phlorizin is a substrate for a glycosidase in intestine which also acts on glucocerebroside and other glycosides and has been reported to block hydrolysis of nitrophenyl glucosides in kidney. However, it was inert toward glucocerebrosidase of placenta.

One series of compounds proved to be *stimulatory* to glucosidase. The series has not as yet been thoroughly studied, but we do know that the aromatic analog of ceramide, N-decanoyl-L-threo-3-phenyl-2-amino-1,3-propanediol, produced 47% more activity at a concentration of 1.2 mM. If this or a similar stimulator can reach the biological site of cerebrosidase action in a patient with Gaucher's disease, there might be sufficient restoration of enzyme activity to slow down the progress of the disease. It is difficult to guess how large a stimulation is needed, but it is clear from enzyme assays of the parents of Gaucher patients that people can get by perfectly well with a considerably depressed level of enzyme. The same has been observed for heterozygotes in other genetic diseases. Perhaps a stimulation of 100 to 200% might produce a normal individual.

The best glucosidase inhibitor was tried in a living system. Hexyl glucosyl sphingosine (HGS) was tested with some cultures of brain tumor cells. Exposure to the inhibitor at a level of 5 μg/ml caused complete loss of enzyme activity without any noticeable effects on the cells. After 7 days of exposure, the rat astrocytoma cells exhibited a 5-fold increase in cellular glucocerebroside, and mouse neuroblastoma cells (type NB41A) exhibited a 6-fold elevation. Thus, we had a model form of Gaucher's disease in these cells (Dawson et al., 1974).

It was also found that the cultured cells could readily absorb labeled glucocerebroside from the medium, a maximal level being achieved within 10 hours. When HGS was included in the medium, the uptake was somewhat slowed, although the ultimate amount of absorbed ^{14}C was not affected. This raises the question of whether glucocerebrosidase is also involved in the absorption process whereby cerebroside is taken up by cells. Of course this question also includes another one: do cells normally take up glucocerebroside from the intercellular fluid? Some preliminary evidence on the second question is available since we found the isolated glial cells, prepared from rat brain, seemed to lack the enzyme which makes glucocerebroside from ceramide and UDP-glucose (Radin et al., 1972a). Isolated neurons did exhibit the enzyme activity, so we concluded that glial cells may obtain their glucocerebroside (or a derived glycolipid) from the adjacent neurons. Also relevant to this question is the conclusion of Dawson and Sweeley (1970) that human red blood cells exchange glucocerebroside with plasma. Thus, it could well turn out that glucocerebrosidase has more than one function, especially in brain.

A similar attempt at inducing Gaucher's disease in cultured cells was made with human fibroblasts in a collaborative study between our laboratory (Kenneth Warren and myself) and the laboratory of Irwin Schafer (and Julia Sullivan and Mary Petrelli). HGS was found to inhibit the human glucosidases that act on nitrophenyl glucoside and on cerebroside. In these cells too (Table VII), the inhibitor caused an accumulation of glucocerebroside but the rate of accumulation was somewhat slower than in the cancerous brain cell cultures. After 28 days of exposure to HGS, the cells exhibited a 2- to 3-fold accumulation of the lipid. There was

Table VII

EFFECTS OF HEXYL GLUCOSYL SPHINGOSINE ON FIBROBLASTS
EXPOSED TO INHIBITOR FOR 28 DAYS

	Cell line			
	ST		PM	
	-HGS	+ HGS	-HGS	+ HGS
Cell dry wt/plate (mg)	6.21	9.42	4.91	5.59
Cerebroside (mg/g dry cells)	0.39	0.80	0.29	0.85
Trihexoside (mg/g dry cells)	1.68	1.96	1.83	2.68
Cholesterol (mg/g dry cells)	24	22	20	21
Total lipid (mg/g dry cells)	166	167	152	166
Protein (mg/g dry cells)	570	570	590	570

also a smaller increase in concentration of GL-3a (ceramide trihexoside) and an increase in dry weight of the cultured cells. The concentrations of cholesterol, total lipid, and total protein were not appreciably affected, indicating that the inhibitor had exerted a rather specific effect.

The finding of an increase in GL-3a agrees with the findings with Gaucher spleens by Kuske and Rosenberg (1972) and by Philippart and Menkes (1967). The increased weight of cells parallels the great increase in spleen size seen in the authentic disease. It does not seem probable that the mere accumulation of a minor lipid component could of itself stimulate growth of an organ or tissue, and the possibility ought to be held in mind that some other functions of cerebrosidase (such as transport) acts to control tissue growth.

The slow rate of glucocerebroside accumulation in the blocked fibroblasts was disappointing but perhaps this is to be expected. In the case of the Gaucher spleen, in the adult form of the disease, accumulation takes many years to become apparent and it is augmented considerably by the role of the spleen in degrading red and white blood cells which daily bring large amounts of glucolipids to be hydrolyzed. Probably our next cell incubation studies should be carried out with the addition of exogenous glucolipids to increase the load rate.

In another study by Kenneth Warren in this laboratory, HGS was injected intraperitoneally into 21 day old rats and its metabolic fate was followed with the aid of ^{14}C in the hexyl group. The amount of radioactivity per gram of tissue, that could be extracted with chloroform-methanol is shown in Fig. 1. (The counting data have been converted for the graph to concentration of inhibitor.) It is evident that the inhibitor went into the organs rapidly but also underwent fairly rapid turnover. Interestingly enough, its highest concentration was found in spleen, and even after 5 days the apparent concentration of HGS was 4.4 µM, which is highly inhibitory *in vitro*.

Analysis of the radioactive lipid extract showed that there were several components. One was a lipid of lower polarity than HGS that we have characterized, by chromatographic matching with standard, as N-hexyl sphingosine. This is the product to be expected if glucocerebrosidase hydrolyzes the glucosidic bond. The rate of hydrolysis is not rapid by *in vitro* standards, but it does occur and the data in Fig. 2 show that the spleen level of HGS decreased 50 % within 1.5 days. This figure also shows the level of hexyl sphingosine, which also dropped fairly rapidly. A small amount of a polar metabolite could also be detected. In liver, this polar metabolite was a somewhat larger component, even higher than the hexyl sphingosine level. In all tissues there was some radioactivity which could not be extracted from the tissue by chloroform-methanol. Perhaps this represents amine that is strongly bound to polyacidic material, and we should have tried extracting with

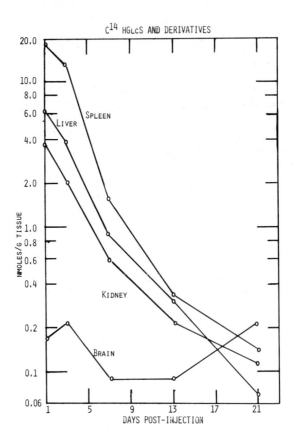

Fig. 1.   *Radioactivity of rat organs after injection of*
^{14}C *HGlcS*.

ammoniacal chloroform-methanol.

This complexity of metabolism of the glucosidase inhibitor is not desirable if one wants to create a live model
of Gaucher's disease, but it is probably unavoidable with
any drug that is administered to an animal. Nonradioactive
HGS was injected into similar rats, at a dosage level of 2
or 5 mg per rat. The higher dose killed 60% of the rats
and slowed the growth of the survivors, but the lower dose
seemed to have no effect on the growth rate. Sacrifice of
the rats from the lower dose after 10 days showed that the
organs did not differ significantly in weight from the
controls (Table VIII). The spleens from the drugged animals

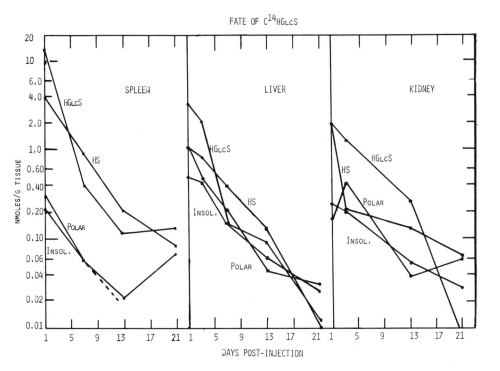

Fig. 2. Radioactivity of rat organs injected with ^{14}C HGlcS (curves show activity of four different radioactive materials in each organ. HGS = N-hexyl sphingosine).

showed a slight increase in total lipid concentration, despite a slight decrease in concentration of cholesterol. The glucocerebroside concentration was appreciably higher than normal, so this encouraged us to try a longer exposure to the inhibitor.

The next group of rats was injected with HGS every 4 or 5 days, with the last injection coming 5 days prior to sacrifice at the 28th day. A lower dosage was used, 1 mg of the hydrochloride per 64 g of body weight. Table IX shows that the growth of the experimental animals was normal but the spleen was appreciably enlarged. The increase in weight was 19% and the tissue seemed darker than normal. The liver too appeared abnormal, somewhat darkened and lumpy in texture. However, an examination of the liver by electron microscopy disclosed no abnormalities.

Table VIII
EFFECT OF INJECTING 2 MG HEXYL GLUCOSYL SPHINGOSINE
INTO 21 DAY OLD RATS; SACRIFICE 10 DAYS LATER

	+ HGS	-HGS
Body weight (g)	104	105
Brain weight (g)	1.57	1.54
Spleen weight (g)	0.37	0.36
Spleen lipid (mg/g)	35.5	31.5
Spleen cholesterol (mg/g)	4.28	4.52
Spleen cerebroside (µg/g)	327	198

Analysis of the spleen showed that the inhibitor had produced a slight decrease in concentrations of lipids, protein, and cholesterol. To our great disappointment, there was only a slight increase in cerebroside level and an assay for glucosidase showed that the activity in spleen was almost normal. Our interpretation of these results is that the rats adapted in some way to the problem of detoxifying the enzyme inhibitor. This adaptation was not detected in our relatively short isotope study of HGS metabolism. It, therefore, looks as though a different inhibitor will be needed in order to generate a long-term model of Gaucher's disease. We are presently preparing a large batch of the aromatic inhibitors mentioned previously in this paper.

Table IX
EFFECT OF PERIODIC INJECTION OF HGS INTO RATS
OVER A 28 DAY PERIOD

	+ HGS	- HGS
Body weight (g)	263	265
Brain weight (g)	1.69	1.67
Spleen weight (g)	0.90	0.76
Spleen total lipid (mg/g)	35.6	39.9
Spleen protein (mg/g)	137	142
Spleen cholesterol (mg/g)	2.52	2.73
Spleen cerebroside (µg/g)	137	121
Spleen trihexoside (µg/g)	20	21
Spleen glucocerebrosidase (nmoles/hr/mg protein)	39	41

We have been carrying out parallel attempts with galactocerebrosidase, using a rat brain preparation, but

haven't reached the stage of animal work for lack of the
rare starting materials. The compound analogous to HGS, N-
hexyl galactosyl sphingosine, was a good inhibitor, but
hardly as effective as with glucosidase. At 0.3 mM, the
inhibition of galactosidase was 68%, so this inhibitor is
only about 1/100th as effective as the glucosyl analog with
glucosidase. However, this degree of inhibition is generally considered useful in biological systems. Curiously,
the galactosyl derivative acted as a mixed-type inhibitor,
suggesting the presence of a second site that could bind
compounds resembling the substrate. A series of aromatic
analogs of ceramide, like the one shown in Table I, proved
to have similar inhibitory power (Arora and Radin, 1972;
Arora *et al.*, 1973).

A comparison of a group of related compounds, all of
them containing 2-hydroxydodecanoic acid bound in amide
linkage is shown in Table X. Comparison of lines 2-4 shows

Table X
INHIBITION OF RAT BRAIN GALACTOSIDASE BY CERAMIDE ANALOGS
(INHIBITORS TESTED AT 0.3 mM)

$$
\begin{array}{c}
3\quad 2\quad 1\\
-CH-CH-CH_2\\
|\quad\ |\quad\ |\\
OH\ NH\ OH\\
|\\
C=O\\
|\\
DL \rightarrow CHOH\\
|\\
C_{10}H_{21}
\end{array}
$$

Substituents	C_2-configuration	C_3-configuration	% inhibition
Formula shown	DL	Erythro	69
Delete OH from fatty acid	DL	Erythro	48
Delete OH from fatty acid	D	Threo	15
Delete OH from fatty acid	L	Threo	17
Deplete OH from position 1	DL	Erythro	16
Delete OH from position 3	DL	Erythro	49
Add P-NO$_2$	DL	Erythro	35

that the DL-erythro structure, which is closest to the
natural configuration of sphingosine, gave better inhibition
than the two threo isomers. The same thing was observed

when a p-nitro group was present, but the nitro group decreased the overall effectiveness (lines 1,7). When either
one of the two hydroxyls on the amino alcohol was deleted,
effectiveness dropped (lines 1,5,6). If the hydroxyl on
the fatty acid was omitted, this too reduced effectiveness
(lines 1,2). Changing the fatty acid chain length, between
10 and 18 carbon atoms, had little effect but replacing the
aromatic ring with a straight chain (that is, using 2-
hydroxydodecanoyl sphingosine) almost completely abolished
the inhibitory effect.

When the most powerful inhibitor was evaluated kinetically, it was found to act as a *non*competitive inhibitor.
Maximal inhibition was 82%, reached at about 0.6 mM. This
is further evidence for the existence of a secondary, mod-
ifying site.

Cerebroside homologs in which the fatty acid was abnormally short were also tried on the theory that they
should bind to the catalytic site but yet prove unhydrolyz-
able. N-acetyl galactosyl sphingosine produced 57% inhibition at 0.3 mM, but kinetic analysis showed that it acted as
a mixed-type inhibitor, like N-hexyl galactosyl sphingosine.

One striking feature of our studies, was the finding
that a variety of compounds strongly resembling the substrate, even with respect to fine points of optical and
isomeric structure, could act as inhibitors at two sites:
some acted only at the catalytic site, some acted only at
some other site, and some acted at both. This was observed
for both gluco- and galactocerebrosidase. I offered this
curiosity to a number of scientific friends and finally
received what seemed like a good insight from Dr. Park
Gerald. He suggested that these enzyme molecules used to be
smaller in the early days of evolution, but at some stage
there was a partial or complete error in gene duplication,
so that the new enzyme consisted of *two* duplicate sections.
Each section contained the same active site, with the same
recognition properties. As the eons of evolutionary modification advanced, one of the sites mutated and lost its
catalytic activity, yet still retained some ability to bind
compounds resembling the substrate.

There is certainly evidence for such gene duplications
in other proteins and the same type of evidence, from pep-
tide mapping, has to be obtained with these enzymes.

The only biological testing with our galactosidase inhibitors has been done by Drs. Joyce Benjamins and John Fitch. Pieces of brain cerebellum from newborn rats were cultured. The development of myelinated fibers was observed. Inhibitors of varying structure and effectiveness were added to the culture medium at age 9-10 days, and the cells were followed for the next 2 to 3 days. The appearance of myelin was blocked by the inhibitors, and the effectiveness of this inhibition was roughly proportional to the *in vitro* effectiveness of these compounds against galactocerebrosidase.

Similar results were obtained when the inhibitors were tested with cultures that had already myelinated somewhat. The most active compounds soon produced demyelination. The nerve axons appeared to be normal but the myelin sheaths became irregular in appearance and eventually turned into balls and disappeared. Some cells, probably glia, became swollen.

Thus, we appear to have produced a syndrome like that seen in the human genetic disorder, globoid leukodystrophy or Krabbe's disease. In this disorder, which strikes infants with fatal intensity, there is a failure to myelinate, with consequent retardation in development and neurological degeneration. Suzuki and Suzuki (1970) have shown that the disease is the result of lack of galactocerebrosidase activity. Some activity *is* present, and more is present in the parents of the children, but evidently there is not enough of the enzyme in the affected children. At present, we can only speculate on the mechanism by which a lack of cerebroside hydrolase prevents myelination.

There are some clues in the literature. One comes from the work of Berthold (1973), who examined the myelin of peripheral nerve fibers microscopically and came to the conclusion that local regions may normally undergo demyelination and remyelination. In other words, it looks as though myelin normally decomposes and reforms in specific areas from time to time. This process may occur in order to reshape the membrane as axonal development proceeds, or to aid the tongue of protruding myelin to envelop the axon. The process by which myelin winds around axons is indeed remarkable, many turns being formed, and in the central nervous system this seems to involve not a wrapping process (like a bandage on a hand) but a protrusion process, by which the outermost layer forces all the inner layers to rotate around the axon. It seems likely that the stiffness

of the membrane, which might well be controlled by cerebroside, would be important to control.

Support for an important role of galactocerebrosidase
in myelin development comes also from a study in our laboratory on the turnover of cerebroside fatty acids. We
found evidence for the existence in rat brain of a fraction
with a half-life shorter than 0.5 days (Hajra and Radin,
1963). The disappearance of radioactive cerebroside acids
presumably depends on cerebrosidase activity.

One unexpected finding in our search for galactosidase
inhibitors came when we examined aliphatic analogs of
ceramide in which a branched methyl group was present at the
2-position. The structure of a series of such compounds
is shown below:

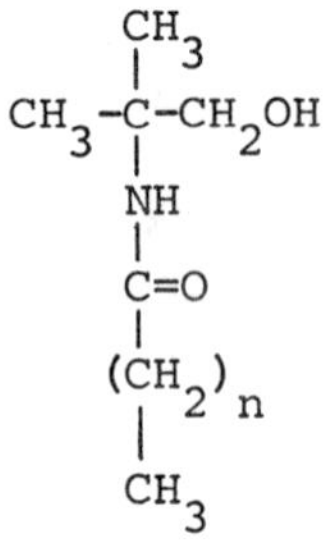

$$
\begin{array}{c}
CH_3 \\
| \\
CH_3-C-CH_2OH \\
| \\
NH \\
| \\
C=O \\
| \\
(CH_2)_n \qquad n=6\text{--}16 \\
| \\
CH_3
\end{array}
$$

The long side chain of sphingosine has been greatly short-
ened and the hydroxyl group in the 3-position has been
deleted. The best of this series, made from decanoic acid,
actually acted as a stimulator for the hydrolase. The amide
worked not only with the rat brain enzyme but equally well
with the human brain enzyme (Radin *et al.*, 1972b). More
importantly, the stimulator also worked with the defective
enzyme that is present in human brain with Krabbe's disease.
Maximal stimulation was 62% with 1 mM amide. Thus, there is
promise in treating such children by a stimulator, as suggested before with reference to Gaucher's disease. It is
also interesting that the substance acted on both the rat
and human enzymes.

We are currently working on the development of inhibitors for the synthetases which make the two cerebrosides.
Perhaps the toxic effects of accumulated cerebroside, particularly in Gaucher's disease, can be minimized by slowing
down the rate of cerebroside synthesis. Chemotherapy might

then consist of administering both a synthetase inhibitor and a hydrolase stimulator.

Summary

Many human genetic disorders involve a deficiency in the activity of a specific enzyme, so that the substrate of the enzyme accumulates in tissues to a toxic level. Most of these disorders cannot be studied in laboratory animals because the defective gene has not yet been observed. It would be useful to develop model forms of these diseases by treating rats with specific inhibitors of the enzyme. We have been attempting to devise such inhibitors for gluco-cerebrosidase (I, involved in Gaucher's disease) and galacto-cerebrosidase (II, involved in Krabbe's disease). Our most effective inhibitor for I was a reduced analog of the sub-strate, N-hexyl-O-glucosyl sphingosine, which acted compet-itively. When the labeled inhibitor was injected intraperi-toneally into rats, it was found to undergo hydrolysis to N-hexyl sphingosine, as well as conversion to polar deriva-tives. Some glucocerebroside accumulation was observed in spleen, but the effect diminished with longer administration of the inhibitor. *In vitro* tests with cultured cells also produced glucocerebroside accumulation. Other inhibitors of I have been made without the glucose moiety: 3-phenyl-2-decylamino-1,3-propanediol and its para-substituted de-rivatives. The amide analogs of the latter are good *non*-competitive inhibitors of II, especially the 2-hydroxy-decanoic acid amide of 3-phenyl-2-amino-1,3-propanediol. These inhibitors have produced a model form of Krabbe's disease in cultured brain explants. Efforts are underway to develop inhibitors of the enzymes which synthesize gluco- and galactocerebroside, since they might block the accumu-lation of these lipids in patients.

References

Arora, R. C., Lin, Y.-N., and Radin, N. S. (1973). *Arch. Biochem. Biophys.* 156, 77.

Arora, R. C., and Radin, N. S. (1972). *J. Lipid Res.* 13, 86.

Berthold, C.-H. (1973). *Neurobiol.* 3, 339.

Bowen, D. M., and Radin, N. S. (1969). *J. Neurochem.* 16, 501.

Dawson, G., Stoolmiller, A. C., and Radin, N. S. (1974). *J. Biol. Chem.* 249, 4634.

Dawson, G., and Sweeley, C. C. (1970). *J. Biol. Chem.* 245, 410.

Erickson, J. S., and Radin, N. S. (1973). *J. Lipid Res.* 14, 133.

Hajra, A. K., and Radin, N. S. (1963). *J. Lipid Res.* 4, 270.

Hyun, J. C., Misra, R. S., Greenblatt, D., and Radin, N. S. (1975). *Arch. Biochem. Biophys.* 166, 382.

Kuske, T. T., and Rosenberg, A. (1972). *J. Lab. Clin. Med.* 80, 523.

Philippart, M., and Menkes, J. H. (1967). *In* "Inborn Disorders of Sphingolipid Metabolism" (S. M. Aronson, and B. W. Volk, eds.), p. 389. Pergamon Press, New York.

Radin, N. S., and Arora, R. C. (1971). *J. Lipid Res.* 12, 256.

Radin, N. S., Brenkert, A., Arora, R. C., Sellinger, O. Z., and Flangas, A. L. (1972a). *Brain Res.* 39, 163.

Radin, N. S., Arora, R. C., Ullman, M. D., Brenkert, A., and Austin, J. (1972b). *Res. Commun. Chem. Pathol. Pharmacol.* 3, 637.

Suzuki, K., and Suzuki, Y. (1970). *Proc. Nat. Acad. Sci.* 66, 302.

Modification of Membrane Glycolipids
By Oncogenic Agents

PETER H. FISHMAN, AND ROSCOE O. BRADY

I. Introduction

One approach to studying cancer is to utilize a model
system in which the various parameters can be controlled.
Animal cells grown in tissue culture represent one such model system. Normal cells grown in culture regulate their
growth and behaviour. The cells grow in oriented monolayers
and, upon reaching a certain population, they stop dividing.
The cessation of growth is due to complex interactions involving cell to cell contacts and requirements for surface
area and nutrients in the growth medium. The processes involved in growth inhibition may be analogous to those involved in the regulation of growth in normal tissues.

In contrast, cells exposed to oncogenic agents grow in
disorganized arrays in culture, pile on top of each other to
form multilayers of cells, and do not stop dividing at high
cell populations. Such cells are said to be transformed.
Transformed cells do not respond to cell to cell contacts,
have reduced requirements for nutrients, can grow without
adhering to the culture vessel, and are malignant in appropriate animals. The transformed cells can be considered
analogous to neoplastic tissues.

For the last several years, research has been directed
toward the surface properties of normal and transformed
cells; because the cell surface is both the point of contact
and the barrier between the cell and its environment, changes
in the cell surface could explain the abnormal behaviour of
transformed cells. This approach has been fruitful and a
number of differences in surface properties have been detected between normal and transformed cells.

More recently, attempts have been made to delineate the biochemical basis of these differences and research has been focused on the complex carbohydrates of the cell surface, especially the sialic acid-containing heteroglycans (Fishman and Brady, 1974). Gangliosides are sialic acid-containing glycosphingolipids that are components of mammalian cell membranes and are highly enriched in plasma membranes. We have been investigating the changes in ganglioside biosynthesis that occur in cultured mouse cells following transformation by oncogenic agents and summarize here our findings which have been carried out in collaboration with several groups at the National Cancer Institute. Modification of membrane gangliosides, as well as neutral glycolipids by oncogenic viruses, has also been reported by other groups and these studies have recently been reviewed (Brady and Fishman, 1974).

II. Ganglioside Metabolism in Normal and Transformed Mouse Cells

A. GANGLIOSIDES IN NORMAL MOUSE CELLS

1. *Ganglioside Composition*

Cultured mouse cells which demonstrate density dependent inhibition of growth and DNA synthesis and which grow to low saturation densities contain a homologous series of gangliosides (Fig. 1). These same four major gangliosides have been found in normal cell lines of Swiss, Balb/c, or AL/N origin, as well as primary and secondary mouse embryo cell cultures (Mora *et al.*, 1969; Brady and Mora, 1970).

2. *Ganglioside Biosynthesis*

The biosynthesis of gangliosides proceeds by the sequential transfer of monosaccharides from sugar nucleotide donors to the growing oligosaccharide chain. Each step is catalyzed by a different glycosyltransferase and the pathway is depicted in Fig. 2. Each of these reactions has been detected in normal mouse cell lines (Fishman *et al.*, 1972). These enzyme activities are routinely assayed in whole cell homogenates but are associated with the membraneous fractions of the cells (Cumar *et al.*, 1970; Fishman *et al.*, 1974a). Incubation conditions are optimized in terms of substrate concentrations, pH, and detergents. In addition, enzyme assays are linear in terms of time and protein content. The reaction products are separated by

Symbol

G_{M3}:   Ceramide-glucose-galactose-N-acetylneuraminic acid

G_{M2}:   Ceramide-glucose-galactose-N-acetylgalactosamine
                                         |
                   N-acetylneuraminic acid

G_{M1}:   Ceramide-glucose-galactose-N-acetylgalactosamine-galactose
                                         |
                   N-acetylneuraminic acid

G_{D1a}:   Ceramide-glucose-galactose-N-acetylgalactosamine-galactose
                                       | |
                   N-acetylneuraminic acid   N-acetylneuraminic acid

Fig. 1. Gangliosides of normal mouse cell lines.

chromatographing the incubation mixtures on small columns of Sephadex G-25 equilibrated with chloroform-methanol-water (60:30:4.5, v/v/v) and collecting the effluents. This procedure effectively separates the radioactive glycolipid products from water soluble radioactive components (Cumar *et al.*, 1970; Fishman *et al.*, 1972). In addition, the reaction products have been identified by thin-layer chromatography on silica gel (Cumar *et al.*, 1970; Fishman *et al.*, 1974a).

B. GANGLIOSIDES IN TRANSFORMED MOUSE CELLS

1. *DNA Virus-Transformed Cells*

In sharp contrast to the complex pattern of gangliosides observed in normal mouse cells, DNA virus-transformed mouse cells have a simplified ganglioside pattern (Mora *et al.*, 1969; Brady and Mora, 1970). The transformed cells have mainly G_{M3}, whereas in the normal cells the majority of the lipid-bound sialic acid is in the higher homologs (Table I). Similar results were observed when normal and SV-40 transformed cells were cultured in media containing radioactive precursors; G_{D1a} was the predominantly labeled ganglioside in normal cells, whereas only G_{M3} was labeled in

107

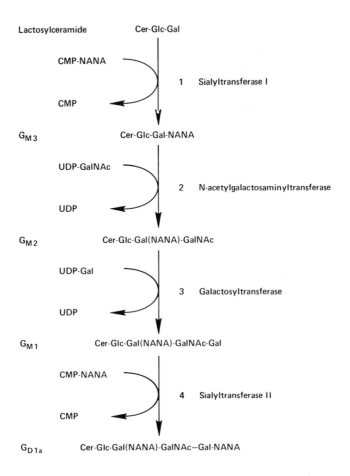

Fig. 2. *Schematic representation of the reactions involved in the biosynthesis of gangliosides.*

the transformed cells (Brady and Mora, 1970).

These results suggested a block in ganglioside biosynthesis; namely, a decrease in UDP-GalNAc: G_{M3} N-acetylgalactosaminyltransferase activity (Fig. 2, reaction 2). Significantly less of this enzyme activity was observed in membrane fractions (Cumar *et al.*, 1970), as well as whole homogenates of DNA virus-transformed cells of Swiss, Balb/c,

Table I

DISTRIBUTION OF GANGLIOSIDES IN NORMAL, SV-40 AND POLYOMA
VIRUS-TRANSFORMED MOUSE CELL LINES

	Gangliosides			
	G_{D1a}	G_{M1}	G_{M2}	G_{M3}
Cell line	% distribution of sialic acid			
Swiss 3T3	36	17	13	34
SV 101	6	6	1	87
PY 11	3	3	1	93
NAL/N	55	23	12	10
SVS-AL/N	12	9	4	75
PY-AL/N	9	6	8	77

Data calculated from Brady and Mora (1970); Mora *et al.*
(1969); Brady *et al.* (1973).

or AL/N origin (Table II). This aberration in ganglioside
metabolism appears to be a rather common occurrence, though
a few exceptions have been observed by us and reported by
others (Brady and Fishman, 1974; Fishman *et al.*, 1973; Mora,
1973). It is also specific as activities of other glycosyltransferases involved in ganglioside biosynthesis (Fig. 2)
were not consistently affected (Fishman *et al.*, 1972).

Table II

UDP-N-ACETYLGALACTOSAMINE: G_{M3} N-ACETYLGALACTOSAMINYL-
TRANSFERASE ACTIVITY IN NORMAL AND DNA TUMOR VIRUS-
TRANSFORMED MOUSE CELL LINES

	Saturation density (Cells/cm^2 x 10^{-5})	Relative activity (As % of normal cells)
Swiss 3T3[a]	0.4	100
SV-101	3.2	13
PY 11	2.0	17
N AL/N	1.0	100
SVS SL/N	3.0	16
PY AL/N	2.4	14
Balb 3T3[b]	0.4	100
SV T$_2$	12.2	23

[a]Data calculated from Fishman *et al.* (1972).
[b]Unpublished observations of P. L. Coleman and P. H. Fishman.
Glycosyltransferase activities were determined on cell homogenates under optimum conditions.

2. *Quantitative Transformation with RNA Virus*

The DNA tumor viruses are well known to transform cells
in culture at relatively low efficiencies and the subsequent
cloning and propagation of transformed cells require a considerable amount of time. It is possible then that the
altered ganglioside metabolism observed in established cloned
transformed cell lines is due to a selection process whereby
only those cells which have low aminosugar transferase activity are transformed and propagated or that a gradual shift
in cell phenotype occurs during the prolonged cultivation of
the transformed cells.

In contrast, RNA tumor viruses under favorable conditions can transform cells virtually quantitatively and very
rapidly. In order to answer the above possible objection,
as well as explore the generality of viral transformation
as it influences ganglioside biosynthesis, we investigated
the transformation of mouse cells by an RNA tumor virus.
Normal Swiss 3T3 cells were infected with a high multiplicity
of Moloney sarcoma virus to ensure rapid and complete transformation. Since the virus stock also contained Moloney
leukemia helper virus, which is nontransforming, Swiss 3T3
cells were also infected with this virus alone. There was a
5-fold reduction in N-acetylgalactosaminyltransferase activity seven days after infection with this virus stock, but
little effect with the nontransforming helper virus alone
(Mora *et al.*, 1973). There was a corresponding reduction in
higher gangliosides in the virally transformed cells (Fig.
3). The levels of the other glycosyltransferases indicated
in Fig. 2 were not decreased (Mora *et al.*, 1973).

3. *A Common Alteration with Different Oncogenic Agents*

It would thus appear that transformation of mouse cells
by both DNA and RNA viruses results in the same specific
change in ganglioside metabolism: a reduction in the activity of a specific aminosugar transferase. However, in the
process of investigation of ganglioside metabolism in other
RNA virus-transformed Balb 3T3 cells, we observed a different pattern (Fig. 4). These cells are a nonproducer line
transformed by the Kirsten strain of murine sarcoma virus
(Aaronson and Weaver, 1971). The major ganglioside in these
cells is G_{M2}. These observations suggested a block in the
galactosyltransferase involved in G_{M1} biosynthesis and there
is a complete absence of this enzymatic activity in these
cells (Fishman *et al.*, 1974a). Again, the effect is specific as other glycosyltransferases are not affected (Table III).

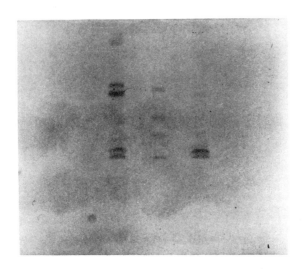

*Fig. 3. Thin-layer chromatography of gangliosides from nor-
mal and Moloney sarcoma virus-transformed Swiss 3T3 cells.
Gangliosides were extracted from the equivalent of 5 mg of
cellular protein, separated by thin-layer chromatography and
silica gel G coated glass plate and detected with resorcinol
spray reagent. From Mora et al. (1973). Left lane - gangliosides from MSV-transformed Swiss 3T3 cells; center lane -
from top to bottom, G_{M3}, G_{M2}, G_{M1}, and G_{D1a}; right lane -
gangliosides from control Swiss 3T3 cells.*

The same block in ganglioside biosynthesis was observed in
other transformed clones isolated by two different selection
procedures (Fishman and Aaronson, unpublished observations).

Recently, we (Coleman et al., 1975) have been able to
demonstrate the same abnormal ganglioside pattern (Fig. 5)
and loss of galactosyltransferase activity (Table IV) in
Balb 3T3 cells transformed by chemical carcinogens and

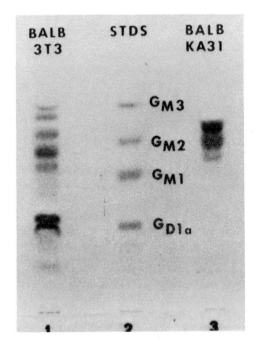

Fig. 4. *Thin-layer chromatogram of gangliosides from normal and Kirsten sarcoma virus-transformed Balb 3T3 cells. Gangliosides corresponding to 5 mg of cellular protein were chromatographed on a thin-layer silica gel G plate and detected with resorcinol spray. From Fishman* et al. *(1974a).*

X-irradiation. The effect of these oncogenic agents is very specific as other ganglioside biosynthetic enzymes are not significantly reduced. Thus, transformation of the same cell line in culture by an RNA virus, different chemical carcinogens, and X-irradiation results in the same modification of membrane gangliosides.

Table III
GLYCOSYLTRANSFERASE ACTIVITIES IN NORMAL AND KIRSTEN
SARCOMA VIRUS-TRANSFORMED BALB 3T3 CELL LINES

Enzyme	Activity in KA31 cells as % of Balb A31 cells
N-acetylgalactosaminyltransferase	103
Galactosyltransferase	0
Sialyltransferase II	92

The clonal Balb 3T3 cell line (clone A31) was transformed
with the Kirsten strain of sarcoma virus and a nonproducer
transformed subclone (KA31) was isolated (Aaronson and Weaver
(1971)). Cell extracts were assayed for the above enzyme
activities (Fishman *et al.* (1974a)).

C. GANGLIOSIDE METABOLISM IN CULTURED MOUSE CELLS UNDER VARIOUS CONDITIONS

1. *Effect of Cell Density and Contact*

Since transformed cells reach higher densities in culture than normal cells and continue to grow after making
intercellular contact, the relationship of these parameters
to ganglioside metabolism was examined. In all of our
studies, normal cells were compared to transformed cells
when both were from exponentially growing sparse cultures.
There were no differences in ganglioside composition where
sparse cultures of normal or transformed cells were compared
to dense cultures. In addition, cell density had no significant effect on the level of the glycosyltransferase activities (Fishman *et al.*, 1972).

Cells that spontaneously transform in culture have
ganglioside compositions and glycosyltransferase activities
similar to normal cells; these include TAL/N and Balb 3T12
which are spontaneously transformed AL/N, and Balb/c cell
lines (Mora *et al.*, 1969; Brady and Mora, 1970; Cumar *et al.*,
1970). Since these cell lines have high saturation densities
in culture, it is unlikely that cell density *per se* affects
ganglioside metabolism.

2. *Growth and Culture Conditions*

Variations in culture medium or pH did not appreciably
influence ganglioside metabolism in normal or transformed
mouse cells (Mora, 1973). Both *in vitro* as well as *in vivo*
selection pressures had little effect on ganglioside metabolism. Thus, when normal cells were continually cultured

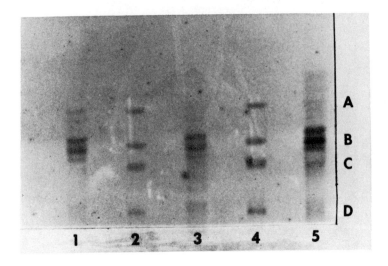

Fig. 5. Thin-layer chromatogram of gangliosides from Balb
3T3 cells transformed by chemical carcinogens and X-irradiation. Gangliosides corresponding to 5 mg of cellular protein were chromatographed on a thin-layer silica gel G plate
and detected with resorcinol spray. From Coleman et al.
(1975). Lane 1 - gangliosides from methylcholanthrene-trans-
formed cells. Lanes 2 and 4 - ganglioside standards G_{M3} (A),
G_{M2} (B), G_{M1} (C), and G_{D1a} (D). Lane 3 - benz-pyrene-trans-
formed cells. Lane 5 - X-irradiation-transformed cells.

under crowded conditions, they did not lose the higher
gangliosides or glycosyltransferase activities. Continuous
passage of normal or virus-transformed mouse cell lines for
over 300 cell generations similarly had no effect. However,
prolonged cultivation of spontaneously transformed cell
lines resulted in losses of higher gangliosides, thus, TAL/N
after 200 tissue culture passages had low galactosyltransferase activity (Fig. 2, reaction 3) and no G_{D1a} or G_{M1}
(Fishman et al., 1973; Hollenberg et al., 1974).

The modified ganglioside metabolism observed in DNA
virus-transformed mouse cells is also stable to in vivo
selection. SVS AL/N cells were injected into syngeneic im-
munosuppressed mice and the induced tumor passed back into
tissue cultures. Even after three repetitions of this
process, the tumor derived cell lines in culture maintained

Table IV
UDP-GALACTOSE: G_{M2} GALACTOSYLTRANSFERASE ACTIVITY IN NORMAL
AND TRANSFORMED BALB 3T3 CELL LINES

Cell line	Transforming agent	Galactosyltransferase activity (pmoles/mg protein/hr)
Balb 3T3, Clone A31	None	511
MC 5.5	Methylcholanthrene	14
BP 117-32	Benz(o)pyrene	30
BP - 8	Benz(o)pyrene	73
R4/Bu	X-irradiation	40
DMBA	Dimethylbenzanthrene	69

Data from Coleman *et al.* (1974) except on DMBA trans-
formant.
The control, Balb 3T3, is a clonal cell line and the transformed cell lines are transformed subclones derived from this
parental line. Activities in cell extracts represent synthesis of G_{M1} from exogenous G_{M2}.

their low N-acetylgalactosaminyltransferase activity (Mora,
1973). When a similar experiment was done with TAL/N cell
line, the tumor derived cell lines maintained their high
aminosugar transferase activity (Fishman and Smith, unpublished).

D. GANGLIOSIDE BIOSYNTHESIS DURING VIRAL INFECTION

DNA tumor viruses have a host range; cells of some
species are permissive for the virus and many become transformed. Other cells are nonpermissive and the virus causes
productive infection whereby new viruses are produced and
released when the host cell undergoes lysis, but tumorigenic
transformation does not occur. Polyoma virus is normally
lytic in mouse cells and rarely transforms; mouse cells are
permissive for SV-40, which is lytic in monkey cells. RNA
leukosis type viruses replicate, but do not transform; however, they are necessary as helper viruses for the replica-
tion and horizontal transmission of the sarcoma viruses.

Cells productively infected with DNA or RNA viruses did
not display the characteristic changes in ganglioside biosynthesis observed in transformed cells. Mouse cells infected with polyoma or Moloney leukemia virus maintained
their high N-acetylgalactosaminyltransferase activity as did
monkey cells infected with SV-40 (Table V). Similarly, Balb
3T3 cells infected with Rauscher leukemia virus had a similar ganglioside composition to uninfected cells (unpublished
observations of Fishman and Aaronson). Thus, viral

Table V

EFFECT OF VIRUS INFECTION ON UDP-GalNAc: G_{M3}
N-ACETYLGALACTOSAMINYLTRANSFERASE ACTIVITY IN CULTURED
MOUSE AND MONKEY CELLS

Cell line	Virus	Days post infection	Transferase activity (% of mock infected cells)
TAL/N[a]	Polyoma	2	131
Swiss 3T3[a]	Polyoma	2	79
Swiss 3T3[b]	MLV	6	80
GMK[c]	SV-40	1	126

[a]Data from Cumar et al. (1970). Activity one day post infection was 129% (TAL/N) and 110% (Swiss 3T3). Cells underwent cytolysis after 4 days.

[b]Data from Mora et al. (1973). Cells were producing Moloney leukemia virus (MLV) when analyzed.

[c]Unpublished observations of P. H. Fishman and L. Couvillon. GMK, green monkey kidney (strain CV-1); activity was 76% at 2 days and 151% at 3 days; cells lysed after 4 days.

transformation, but not viral infection, is associated with altered ganglioside biosynthesis.

III. Modulation of Transformation and Ganglioside Biosynthesis

A. FLAT PHENOTYPE REVERTANTS

The experimental evidence indicates that cells transformed by a variety of oncogenic agents contain less of the more polar gangliosides due to specific blocks in ganglioside biosynthesis. If this phenomenon is associated with the transformed phenotype, modulation of the expression of transformation should result in a modulation of ganglioside biosynthesis.

Phenotypic revertants can be selected from virus-transformed cells by various techniques (Pollack et al., 1968; Smith et al., 1971) and these revertants, though retaining the virus genome, will have acquired many of the phenotypic properties of normal cells, such as low saturation density, in culture. Flat revertants isolated from SV-40 transformed mouse cells contained a ganglioside pattern and N-acetylgalactosaminyltransferase activity similar to normal cells (Table VI). Flat polyoma revertants which were

Table VI
UDP-N-ACETYLGALACTOSAMINE: G_{M3} N-ACETYLGALACTOSAMINYL-
TRANSFERASE ACTIVITY IN NORMAL SV-40 TRANSFORMED AND
FLAT REVERTANT MOUSE CELL LINES

Cell line	Saturation density (cells/cm^2 x 10^{-5})	Transferase activity (as % of control cells)
Swiss 3T3	0.4	100
SV-40 transformed	3.2	30
Flat revertant	0.13	135
Balb/c 3T3[b]	0.5	100
SV-40 transformed	4.2	38
Flat revertant	0.3	132

[a]Data calculated from Mora et al. (1969) (Table III,
experiment number 1).
[b]Data calculated from Fishman et al. (1973).

phenotypically and genotypically heterogenous (Pollack et al., 1970) showed a partial restoration of ganglioside biosynthesis (Mora et al., 1971). These experiments suggested that there is a coordinate link between the biochemical change and the expression of transformation.

B. TEMPERATURE-SENSITIVE MUTANT VIRUSES

A second way to modulate the transformed phenotype is to transform cells with thermosensitive mutant viruses. When grown at the permissive temperature, the cells will be transformed; when grown at the nonpermissive temperatures, the cells will return to the normal phenotype. Although mouse cells transformed by thermosensitive viruses are not available, we did examine a SV-40 transformed Swiss 3T3 cell line that was temperature-sensitive for a host cell function involved in transformation (Renger and Basilico, 1972). In these cells there was no modulation of ganglioside metabolism by culture temperature (Mora, 1973). This may be a consequence of the mutation being in the cell and not the virus.

We did observe a modulation of ganglioside synthesis in a second thermosensitive cell line. Newborn rat kidney cells (NRK) contain only G_{M3}. When transformed by various RNA sarcoma viruses, there is a decrease in G_{M3} due to reduced sialyltransferase activity (Fig. 2, reaction 1) as indicated in Table VII.

Table VII

LEVELS OF GANGLIOSIDE G_{M3} AND CMP-SIALIC ACID:
LACTOSYLCERAMIDE SIALYLTRANSFERASE ACTIVITY IN NORMAL AND
RNA VIRUS-TRANSFORMED RAT CELLS

Cell line	Morphology	G_{M3} (nmol/mg protein)	Sialyltransferase (% of normal)
NRK	Normal	1.99	100
MSV-NRK	Transformed	–	69
WSV-NRK	Transformed	1.08	50
KiSV-NRK	Transformed	1.10	30

Unpublished data of P. H. Fishman, S. A. Aaronson and R. Bassin.

MSV, Moloney sarcoma virus; WSV, Wooley monkey sarcoma virus; KiSV, Kirsten sarcoma virus; NRK, newborn rat kidney.

Dr. Stuart Aaronson has provided us with NRK cells transformed by a temperature-sensitive mutant of KiSV (Scolnick *et al.*, 1972). When grown at 39°C, these cells behave as normal cells; at 31°C, the cells are transformed. The G_{M3} content of these cells is also modulated by the growth temperature, being lower at the transforming temperature similar to that found in the wild type transformants. Sialyltransferase activity is similarly affected (Table VIII).

Table VIII

EFFECT OF GROWTH TEMPERATURE ON CMP-SIALIC ACID:
LACTOSYLCERAMIDE SIALYLTRANSFERASE ACTIVITY IN NORMAL AND
KIRSTEN SARCOMA VIRUS-TRANSFORMED RAT CELLS

Cell line	Sialyltransferase activity 31°C	39°C
	(% of normal cells)	
NRK	100	100
KiSV-NRK	44	28
TS-NRK	40	154

Unpublished data of P. H. Fishman and S. A. Aaronson.

NRK, newborn rat kidney; KiSV, Kirsten sarcoma virus; TS, thermosensitive mutant of KiSV. Cells were grown at 31°C and 39°C and homogenates assayed for sialyltransferase activity.

C. INDUCTION OF GLYCOLIPID BIOSYNTHESIS

In collaboration with Dr. Ernst Freese of our institute, we have developed a third model system to correlate changes in the expression of cell phenotype with ganglioside metabolism. HeLa, a human tumor cell line, undergoes marked morphological changes when cultured in the presence of

certain short chain fatty acids (Ginsburg *et al.*, 1973).
When exposed to millimolar concentrations of sodium butyrate,
HeLa cells will stop growing, extend long processes, and
become more fibroblastoid (Fig. 6). Under these conditions,
the content of G_{M3} is elevated 3-4-fold due to a specific
increase (12-20-fold) in sialyltransferase I activity
(Fishman *et al.*, 1974b). There are no substantial changes
in other glycolipids or glycosyltransferases (Table IX) and
G_{M3}-sialidase activity remains unchanged (Tallman, Fishman,
and Henneberry, unpublished observations).

The changes in sialyltransferase I activity and morphology are time dependent and depend on RNA and protein
synthesis (Fishman *et al.*, 1974b; Simmons *et al.*, 1975).
Thus, the increase in glycolipid biosynthesis is due to
enzyme induction, which is reversed by removal of the butyrate. Changes in enzyme activity always precede changes in
cell shape. Similarly, only those fatty acids (butyrate,
pentanoate, and propionate) that induce sialyltransferase
activity cause changes in cell morphology. We are still
investigating the mechanisms for this induction of ganglioside biosynthesis and its relationship to changes in cell
morphology. However, the present data indicates that ganglioside biosynthesis is correlated with the expression of cell
shape which resembles the reversal of cell transformation.

IV. Molecular Basis for Altered Ganglioside Biosynthesis

A. AT THE LEVEL OF ENZYME ACTIVITY

Our investigations indicate that it is necessary that
the viral genome be integrated into the DNA of the host cell
in order to produce the observed changes in ganglioside pattern and synthesis in virus-transformed cells. In the case
of cells transformed by chemical carcinogens and X-irradiation, modification of the host cell DNA may be necessary
for these changes to occur. Alternatively, the same modification of glycolipid biosynthesis observed in these transformed subclones of Balb 3T3, as well as Kirsten sarcoma
virus-transformants, may be related to the activation of a
latent virus. The principal question that has to be an-
swered is how the insertion of new (viral) information into
the host cell or modification (or activation) of host cell
DNA results in the expression of an alteration in membrane
glycolipids.

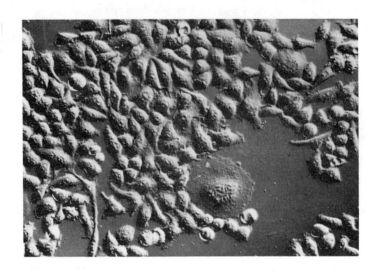

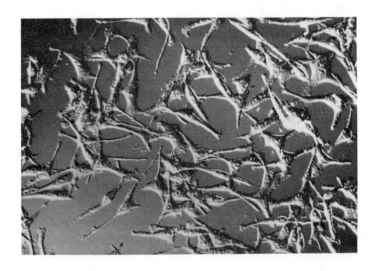

Fig. 6. Effect of butyrate on HeLa cells. HeLa cells were grown for 12 hours in standard medium (top) and in medium supplemented with 5 MM sodium butyrate (bottom). Photomicrographs are 160 X.

There are several possibilities. The simplest would be that the new genetic information codes for an inhibitor specific for the appropriate glycosyltransferase. Thus, DNA virus-transformed mouse cells would contain an inhibitor of N-acetylgalactosaminyltransferase. No inhibitor (or absence of an enzyme activator) was detected in microsomal

Table IX

EFFECT OF BUTYRATE ON GLYCOLIPID BIOSYNTHESIS IN HELA CELLS

Glycolipid concentrations	% of control	Glycosyltransferase activity	% of control
cer-glc	173	β-glucosyltransferase	97
cer-glc-gal	110	β-galactosyltransferase	67
cer-glc-gal-gal	119	α-galactosyltransferase	125
cer-glc-gal-NAN	351	α-sialyltransferase	1311

Data calculated from Fishman et al. (1974b) and Simmons et al. (1974). HeLa cells were cultured for 24 hours in normal or 5 mM butyrate supplemented medium. The cells were then analyzed for glycolipids and glycosyltransferase activities which are expressed as the percent found in control cells. Each glycosyltransferase catalyzes the addition of the termined monosaccharide on the corresponding glycolipid.

fractions (Cumar et al., 1970) or in whole homogenates of SV-40 transformed cells (Mora et al., 1971). Similarly, when whole homogenates of normal and Moloney sarcoma virus-transformed Swiss 3T3 cells were mixed and assayed, the expected activity of N-acetylgalactosaminyltransferase was obtained (Mora et al., 1973). Mixing of cell extracts from normal Balb 3T3 cells and cells transformed by chemical carcinogens and X-irradiation had no effect on galactosyltransferase activity (Table X).

These experiments indicate that there is no readily detectable enzyme inhibitor in transformed cells. However, the possibility that there is a membrane bound inhibitor cannot be excluded. When SVS-AL/N and TAL/N cells (the latter have aminosugar transferase activity) were grown under common medium, there was no evidence for a diffusible inhibitor secreted from the SV-40 transformed cells or a diffusible enzyme activator from the TAL/N cells (Mora et al., 1971). However, when these cells were grown in mixed culture, the activity of N-acetylgalactosaminyltransferase was significantly less than expected (Table XI). Although equal numbers of each cell type were seeded in each experiment, when the actual ratio of cells was determined at harvest in experiment two, the distribution was 62% TAL/N and 38% SVS SL/N (Mora et al., 1971). Thus, the degree of

121

Table X

THE EFFECT OF MIXING CELL EXTRACTS FORM NORMAL AND
TRANSFORMED BALB 3T3 MOUSE CELL LINES ON UDP-GALACTOSE:
G_{M2} GALACTOSYLTRANSFERASE ACTIVITY

| | Galactosyltransferase activity | | | |
| Cell line | Separate | Mixed | Expected | % of expected |
	(pmol/mg protein/hr			
A31	535	–	–	–
BP-8	60	327	298	110
MCS-5	14	242	275	88
R_4/B	49	286	292	98

Data from Coleman *et al.* (1974). Extracts of each cell
line were assayed for galactosyltransferase activity separately and admixed with an equivalent amount of protein from
the normal A31 cell line. Activities represent synthesis of
G_{M1} from exogenous G_{M2}.

inhibition may even be greater than that calculated in Table
XII. The underlying mechanism for this observed inhibition
is unknown, but is worth pursuing as the effect appears to
be specific. When UDP-galactose: G_{M2} galactosyltransferase

Table XI

UDP-N-ACETYLGALACTOSAMINE: G_{M3} N-ACETYLGALACTOSAMINYL-
TRANSFERASE ACTIVITY IN SEPARATE AND MIXED CULTURES OF
SPONTANEOUSLY AND SV-40 TRANSFORMED MOUSE CELLS

| | N-acetylgalactosaminyltransferase activity (cpm/mg protein)[c] | | |
Cell culture	Exp. 1[a]	Exp. 2[a]	Exp. 3[b]
TAL/N	8,370	23,205	29,000
SVS SL/N	1,536	66	1,147
Mixed	2,736	8,823	6,747
Expected activity	4,953	11,636	15,074
% Inhibition	45	24	55

[a]Data from Mora *et al.* (1973). In both experiments equal
numbers of each cell line were plated separately or together
(1/2 of the numbers plated separately). In experiment 1,
cells were harvested after 3 days and in experiment 2, after
5 days. Cells in either experiment were not confluent. In
experiment 1, UDP-GalNAc and G_{M3} concentrations were 1/2
those in experiment 2.
[b]Observations of P. H. Fishman and L. Couvillon. Equal
numbers of cells were plated and harvested after 3 days when
the cells were confluent. Enzyme activity was assayed with
optimum concentrations of substrates.
[c]Activity represents synthesis of G_{M2} from exogenous G_{M3};
incubation times were 3 hours for experiment 1 and 2, and 2
hours for experiment 3.

activity was determined in the mixture culture from experiment three, there was no evidence for enzyme inhibition.

Table XII

PROPERTIES OF UDP-N-ACETYLGALACTOSAMINE: G_{M3}
N-ACETYLGALACTOSAMINYLTRANSFERASE ACTIVITY IN NORMAL AND
SV-40 TRANSFORMED BALB 3T3 MOUSE CELLS

Enzyme property	Cell line	
	Balb 3T3	SVT 2
Km, UDP-GalNAC (µM)	85	105
Km, G_{M3} (mM)	0.69	0.65
pH optimum	7.4	7.2
V_{max} (nmol/mg protein/hr)	3.3	0.77

Data of P. L. Coleman and P. H. Fishman.

B. AT THE LEVEL OF DNA

A second possibility is that the viral genome integrates at a site in the host cell DNA, that which prevents transcription of the gene coding for the appropriate transferase, or results in synthesis of a less active enzyme. In the case of Balb 3T3 cells transformed by chemicals or X-irradiation, this critical site could be modified or be the focus of a latent virus. Several lines of evidence argue against this possibility. Viral DNA appears to be integrated during lytic infection of monkey cells with SV-40 (Hirai and Defendi, 1972) and of mouse cells with polyoma (Babiuk and Hudson, 1972) and under these conditions there was no observable decrease in ganglioside biosynthesis (Table V). There is integrated viral DNA in the flat revertant cell lines which is partially functioning as the revertants are T-antigen positive (T-antigen is a virus-specific nuclear antigen). Yet, these revertant cell lines are able to synthesize the higher ganglioside homologs. In the rat cells transformed by a thermosensitive RNA virus, viral DNA is integrated at both the permissive and nonpermissive temperatures, but transformation and reduced G_{M3} biosynthesis is only expressed at the lower temperature. Finally, kinetic analysis of the residual glycosyltransferase activities in the transformed mouse cells (Tables XII and XIII) indicated that these enzymatic activities were similar to that in untransformed mouse cells. Thus, the presence of newly expressed genetic information in the transformed cell does not lead to the production of modified glycosyltransferase enzymes.

123

Table XIII

PROPERTIES OF UDP-GALACTOSE: G_{M2} GALACTOSYLTRANSFERASE
ACTIVITY IN NORMAL AND TRANSFORMED BALB 3T3 MOUSE CELL LINES

Cell line	Enzyme property		
	K_m (UDP-Gal) (M)	K_m (G_{M2}) (M)	T 1/2 at 51°C (min)
Normal			
A31	300	9	1.6
Transformed			
BP-8	310	30	1.7
MC5-5	350	12	1.4
R_4/B	280	20	1.9

Data from Coleman *et al.* (1974). See Table IV for a
description of the cell lines and the levels of galactosyltransferase activity in them.

C. AT THE LEVEL OF PROTEIN SYNTHESIS

A third possibility is that the transformed cells contain a specific repressor which interferes with the synthesis of the affected glycosyltransferase at the level of
translation. Thus, SV-40, polyoma, and Moloney sarcoma virus would produce a common repressor which would prevent the
translation of the messenger RNA that codes for N-acetylgalactosaminyltransferase. Presumably, thermosensitive mutant viruses code for a thermolabile polypeptide which is
necessary for the expression of transformation. Thus, in
the TS-NRK cells, this heat sensitive protein could be a
repressor for the synthesis of sialyltransferase I. Our
studies with the HeLa cells indicates that glycolipid biosynthesis can be induced and is presumably under some type
of regulatory control. A likely mechanism would be a repressor protein that is inactivated or no longer synthesized in response to butyrate. A tenable model for transformation would be that oncogenic agents interfere with
normal cell regulatory mechanisms. In the case of glycolipid biosynthesis, they lead to the continual presence of a
cellular repressor which prevents the synthesis of key
glycosyltransferases.

Summary

Normal mouse cells contain a homologous series of
gangliosides. Tumorigenic transformation by a variety of
oncogenic agents including DNA and RNA viruses, chemical
carcinogens, and X-irradiation results in a loss of the more

124

polar gangliosides due to specific blocks in ganglioside
biosynthesis. The decreased glycosyltransferase activities
observed in these transformed mouse cells appear to be associated with the transformation process and not a secondary
consequence of the altered growth properties of transformed
cells. The generality of this phenomenon and the altered
ganglioside metabolism observed during the mass transformation of cell cultures with an RNA virus indicates that
these changes are not due to selection of preexisting cells
that possess reduced glycosyltransferase activities. In
the case of virus-transformed cells, the changes in ganglioside biosynthesis are associated with viral transformation
and not viral infection. In several instances, modulation
of the host cell phenotype results in an expression or suppression of ganglioside biosynthesis in parallel with the
expression or suppression of the more normal phenotype.
The discovery of this modification of membrane glycolipids
by oncogenic agents may be an important implement to cancer
research.

References

Aaronson, S. A., and Weaver, C. A. (1971). *J. Gen. Virol.*
13, 245.
Babuik, L. A., and Hudson, J. B. (1972). *Biochem.*
Biophys. Res. Commun. 47, 111.
Brady, R. O., and Fishman, P. H. (1974). *Biochim. Biophys.*
Acta 355, 121.
Brady, R. O., Fishman, P. H., and Mora, P. T. (1973).
Federation Proceedings 32, 102.
Brady, R. O., and Mora, P. T. (1970). *Biochim. Biophys.*
Acta 218, 308.
Coleman, P. L., Fishman, P. H., Brady, R. O., and Todaro,
G. J. (1975). *Biol. Chem,* 250, 55.
Cumar, F. A., Brady, R. O., Kolodny, E. H., McFarland, V.
W., and Mora, P. T. (1970). *Proc. Natl. Acad. Sci.*
USA 67, 757.
Dijong, I., Mora, P. T., and Brady, R. O. (1971). *Biochem.*
10, 4039.
Fishman, P. H., and Brady, R. O. (1974). *In* "Biological
Roles of Sialic Acid" (A. Rosenberg and C. L. Schen-
grund, eds.). Plenum Press, New York, in press.
Fishman, P. H., Brady, R. O., Bradley, R. M., Aaronson, S.
A., and Todaro, G. J. (1974a). *Proc. Natl. Acad.*
Sci. USA 71, 298.
Fishman, P. H., Simmons, J. L., Brady, R. O., and Freese,
E. (1974b). *Biochem. Biophys. Res. Commun.* 59, 292.

Fishman, P. H., Brady, R. O., and Mora, P. T. (1973). *In* "Tumor Lipids: Biochemistry and Metabolism" (R. Wood, ed.), p. 250. American Oil Chemists' Society Press, Champaign, Illinois.

Fishman, P. H., McFarland, V. W., Mora, P. T., and Brady, R. O. (1972). *Biochem. Biophys. Res. Commun.* 48, 48.

Ginsburg, E., Solomon, D., Sreevalsan, T., and Freese, E. (1973). *Proc. Natl. Acad. Sci. USA* 70, 2457.

Hirai, K., and Defendi, V. (1972). *J. Virol.* 9, 705.

Hollenberg, M. D., Fishman, P. H., Bennett, V., and Cuatrecasas, P. (1974). *Proc. Natl. Acad. Sci. USA* 71, in press.

Mora, P. T. (1973). *In* "Membrane-Mediated Information" (P. W. Kent, ed.), p. 64, v. 1. Medical and Technical Publishing Company, Ltd. Lancaster.

Mora, P. T., Fishman, P. H., Bassin, R. H., Brady, R. O., and McFarland, V. W. (1973). *Nature New Biol.* 245, 226.

Mora, P. T., Cumar, F. A., and Brady, R. O. (1971). *Virology* 46, 60.

Mora, P. T., Brady, R. O., Bradley, R. M., and McFarland, V. W. (1969). *Proc. Natl. Acad. Sci. USA* 63, 1290.

Pollack, R. E., Wolman, S., and Vogel, A. (1970). *Nature* 228, 938.

Pollack, R. E., Green, H., and Todaro, G. J. (1968). *Proc. Natl. Acad. Sci. USA* 60, 126.

Renger, H. C., and Basilico, C. (1972). *Proc. Natl. Acad. Sci. USA* 69, 109.

Scolnick, E. M., Stephenson, J. R., and Aaronson, S. A. (1972). *J. Virology* 10, 653.

Simmons, J. L., Fishman, P. H., Freese, E., and Brady, R. O. (1975). *J. Cell Biol.* 66, 414.

Smith, H. S., Scher, C. D., and Todaro, G. J. (1971). *Virology* 44, 359.

Dietary Regulation of Lipid
Metabolism

DALE R. ROMSOS, AND GILBERT A. LEVEILLE

I. Introduction

Lipid metabolism and its regulation has been a focal
point of much research recently. In this review, we will
provide a synopsis of our studies on the effect of diet on
the control of lipid metabolism. These studies have been
conducted using three species, the rat, pig, and chick,
known to differ in certain aspects of lipid metabolism. For
example, the pig synthesizes virtually all of its fatty acids
in adipose tissue (O'Hea and Leveille, 1969; Romsos et al.,
1971), the liver is the predominant lipogenic organ in the
chick (Leveille et al., 1968; O'Hea and Leveille, 1968) and
the rat is intermediate synthesizing fatty acids in both
liver and adipose tissue (Leveille, 1967a). Our choice of
illustrations is not meant to imply that these are the only
dietary factors involved in the control of lipid metabolism,
but rather it is an attempt to demonstrate that various
dietary ingredients may function at different control points
and that in some cases there are species-specific responses
to these dietary ingredients. We hope that our use of these
illustrations will stimulate thought and encourage further
research to clarify those many areas which remain ambiguous.

II. Dietary Fat

Many studies have dealt with the effect of fasting or
fat feeding on the control of lipogenesis. It is clear that
dietary fat influences fatty acid synthesis in rats, pigs,
and chicks (Table I). The early observations that plasma-
free fatty acid and hepatic long chain acyl CoA levels were
inversely correlated with the rate of hepatic fatty acid
synthesis suggested that these metabolites might act as inhibitors of fatty acid synthesis. However, the physiological

Table I

INFLUENCE OF DIETARY FAT ON LIPOGENESIS IN RATS, PIGS AND CHICKS[a]

	Species	Tissue	Dietary fat, %	
			1-2	10-14
In vitro FAS	Rat	Liver	100[b]	32
		Adipose	100	44
	Pig	Adipose	100	53
	Chick	Liver	100	29
Malic enzyme	Rat	Liver	100	32
		Adipose	100	38
	Pig	Adipose	100	71
	Chick	Liver	100	52

[a]From Wiley and Leveille (1973); Allee et al. (1971); Yeh et al. (1970). Animals were fed their respective diets for 3-5 weeks.
[b]Relative rate of glucose-^{14}C conversion to fatty acids in vitro and of malic enzyme activity.

significance of long chain acyl CoA derivatives as controllers of lipogenesis was subsequently questioned since these metabolites were shown to be strong detergents with nonspecific effects on many enzymes (Srere, 1965; Dorsey and Porter, 1968). Recently, Goodridge has demonstrated that long chain acyl CoA derivatives do exert specific effects on acetyl CoA carboxylase (Fig. 1). He demonstrated that palmitoyl CoA specifically inhibited acetyl CoA carboxylase without influencing the activity of other lipogenic enzymes and that this effect could be reversed by addition of albumin to the mixture (Goodridge, 1972). This reversal of inhibition ruled out a detergent action of palmitoyl CoA.

We fasted or fed high fat diets to chicks to ascertain the influence of these dietary alterations on plasma-free fatty acid levels, hepatic acyl CoA levels, and the rate of fatty acid synthesis. The in vivo rate of fatty acid synthesis was markedly depressed by addition of fat to the diet or by a short-term fast (Tables II and III). Conversely, plasma-free fatty acid levels were increased as were hepatic long chain acyl CoA levels when chicks were fed high fat diets or fasted. Free CoA participates in the citrate cleavage reaction to form acetyl CoA. Feeding the high fat diet or fasting decreased the hepatic-free CoA levels (Tables II and III). Thus, CoA derivatives may be involved in the control of fatty acid synthesis at several points. As discussed, long chain acyl CoA derivatives specifically inhibit

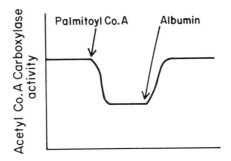

*Fig. 1. Inhibition of chick liver acetyl coA carboxylase
activity by palmitoyl CoA. Acetyl CoA carboxylase activity
was restored to its original level by increasing the albumin
concentration in the medium. From Goodridge (1972).*

acetyl CoA carboxylase; they also inhibit citrate transport
from the mitochondria (Halperin *et al.*, 1972). Citrate is
not only the substrate for fatty acid synthesis, but also

Table II
DIETARY FAT, HEPATIC FATTY ACID SYNTHESIS AND METABOLITE
LEVELS IN THE CHICK[a]

	Dietary fat, %	
	2	26
In vivo FAS[b]	4.3 ± 1.1	0.2 ± 0.03
Plasma FFA, μeq/l	496 ± 16	794 ± 80
Hepatic		
Free CoA[c]	78 ± 10	49 ± 6
Acetyl CoA	25 ± 6	15 ± 2
Acyl CoA	20 ± 3	70 ± 6

[a]From Yeh and Leveille (1971). Diets were fed for 3 weeks.
[b]% of acetate-^{14}C dose recovered in liver fatty acids.
[c]Nanomoles of metabolite per gram of liver.

is an activator of acetyl CoA carboxylase. Changes in long
chain acyl CoA levels would also affect the availability of
free CoA for the citrate cleavage reaction.

Table III
EFFECT OF A SHORT-TERM FAST ON HEPATIC FATTY ACID
SYNTHESIS AND METABOLITE LEVELS IN THE CHICK[a]

	Hours fasted	
	0	2
In vivo FAS[b]	4.6 ± 0.4	0.3 ± 0.1
Plasma FFA, µeq/l	412 ± 52	828 ± 83
Hepatic		
Free CoA[c]	63 ± 4	43 ± 4
Acetyl CoA	26 ± 6	9 ± 1
Acyl CoA	11 ± 1	83 ± 9

[a]From Yeh and Leveille (1971). Diets were fed for 3 weeks.
[b]% of acetate-^{14}C dose recovered in liver fatty acids.
[c]Nanomoles of metabolite per gram of liver.

While a major effort has been directed toward an understanding of the role of the quantity of dietary fat consumed
on the control of lipid metabolism, there has also been an
interest in the influence of composition of the dietary fatty
acids on lipogenesis. Musch *et al.* (1974) have recently
provided evidence that polyunsaturated fatty acids are more
effective than monoenoic fatty acids in reducing the activity
of lipogenic enzymes in rat liver (Table IV). Diets containing methyl linolenate reduced the activity of lipogenic

Table IV
INFLUENCE OF METHYL OLEATE AND METHYL LINOLENATE ON
LIPOGENIC ENZYME ACTIVITY IN RAT LIVER[a]

	Dietary fat		
	None	Methyl oleate	Methyl linolenate
Glucose-6-phosphate dehydrogenase	263 ± 66	194 ± 51	146 ± 41
Fatty acid synthetase	49 ± 9	52 ± 8	36 ± 5
Malic enzyme	210 ± 8	205 ± 51	143 ± 27

[a]From Musch *et al.* (1974). Diets fed for 7 days. Methyl
esters supplied 4% calories. Results expressed as units per
mg protein.

enzymes, including glucose-6-phosphate dehydrogenase, fatty
acid synthetase and malic enzyme, to a greater extent than
did diets containing methyl oleate. In fact, addition of
methyl oleate to the fat-free diet did not depress the activity of lipogenic enzymes.

Few studies have dealt with the mechanisms by which polyunsaturated fatty acids might exert their effects, distinct from those of saturated fatty acids. Numerous studies have compared the efficacy of polyunsaturated fatty acids and highly saturated fatty acids in depressing lipogenesis. We postulated that one mechanism whereby such dietary treatments might influence metabolism may be related to the efficiency of absorption of the specific fats. We fed tripalmitin and safflower oil to chicks (Table V) and observed

Table V

DIETARY FAT SOURCE AND HEPATIC LIPOGENESIS IN CHICKS[a]

	Diet		
	Fat-free	Tripalmitin	Safflower oil
In vitro FAS[b]	1573 ± 118	1399 ± 205	878 ± 91
Malic enzyme[c]	213 ± 22	172 ± 21	138 ± 12
Citrate cleavage enzyme[c]	147 ± 12	134 ± 8	79 ± 7
Plasma FFA, μeg/l	720 ± 24	640 ± 85	1388 ± 140
Apparent fat absorpion, %	-	45 ± 2	94 ± 2

[a]From Romsos et al. (1975a). Diets fed for 5 days and contained 10% fat.

[b]Nmoles glucose-^{14}C converted to fatty acids per 100 mg liver slice per 2 hr.

[c]Nmoles substrate converted to produce per mg protein per minute at 25°.

that the addition of safflower oil to the fat-free diet significantly depressed the in vitro rate of fatty acid synthesis and lipogenic enzyme activity. Dietary tripalmitin was much less effective. However, less than half of the dietary tripalmitin was absorbed (Table V). Undoubtedly, this was a major factor in the reduced response of the chick to this lipid. Clearly, factors other than efficiency of fat absorption are also involved; however, this experiment does illustrate that estimates of factors, such as nutrient absorption, are crucial components of studies where the treatments involve different diets.

III. Dietary Protein

The interrelationship between dietary fat and carbohydrate in the control of lipid metabolism has received major emphasis. Few studies have been directed at the role of dietary protein in the control of lipogenesis. Interpretation of studies involving dietary protein, as well as dietary fat or carbohydrate, is confounded since variation in the quantity of one dietary ingredient is at the expense of another dietary ingredient. Increasing the level of dietary protein has been reported to depress fatty acid synthesis in rats, pigs, and chicks (Table VI). In these

Table VI
EFFECT OF DIETARY PROTEIN ON LIPOGENESIS IN RATS, PIGS AND CHICKS[a]

	Species	Tissue	Dietary protein, %	
			9-12	36-48
In vitro FAS	Rat	Adipose	100	38
	Pig	Adipose	100	20
	Chick	Liver	100	18

[a]From Leveille (1967b); O'Hea *et al.* (1970); and Yeh and Leveille (1969). Results expressed as relative rate of fatty acid synthesis *in vitro*.

studies, changes in dietary protein were at the expense of dietary carbohydrate. Thus, the changes observed might have resulted from an increase in dietary protein or from a decrease in dietary carbohydrate. We will discuss several studies designed to examine the influence of dietary protein on hepatic lipogenesis in the chick and also present evidence suggesting that dietary protein and fat depresses fatty acid synthesis through different mechanisms.

Yeh and Leveille (1969) studied the influence of protein quantity, as well as protein quality, on hepatic lipogenesis in chicks. Chicks fed a diet containing 18% protein, rather than 12% protein, exhibited more than a 50% depression in the *in vitro* rate of fatty acid synthesis (Table VII). To study the influence of protein quality on hepatic fatty acid synthesis in the chick, graded levels of lysine were added to a diet containing sesame meal (deficient in lysine) as the protein source. The effective protein levels were calculated according to the amount of lysine added. The rate of fatty acid synthesis was similar for the 2 groups of chicks fed 18% protein with an effective protein level of either 8% or 18% (Table VII). This study demonstrated that protein level, rather than protein quality influenced hepatic lipogenesis in the chick. Body fat followed the same trend as fatty acid synthesis, being depressed by increasing protein levels (Table VII).

Table VII
INFLUENCE OF DIETARY PROTEIN LEVEL ON FATTY ACID SYNTHESIS
IN CHICK LIVER[a]

	Group		
	1	2	3
Dietary protein, %	12	18	18
Effective protein, %[b]	12	8	18
Fatty acid synthesis[c]	1474 ± 101	652 ± 46	668 ± 88
Body fat, %	15 ± 1	11 ± 1	10 ± 1

[a]From Yeh and Leveille (1969). Diets fed for 3 weeks.
[b]The effective protein level was calculated according to the amount of lysine added to the lysine-deficient basal diet.
[c]Nanomoles acetate-^{14}C converted to fatty acid per 100 mg tissue per 2 hr.

In another study, chicks were allowed access to a protein-adequate diet for 2 days and then a protein-free diet for the third day of a 3 day cycle (Leveille and Yeh, 1972). This feeding schedule continued for 8 cycles and markedly influenced hepatic fatty acid synthesis and lipogenic enzyme activity (Fig. 2). Conversion of glucose-U-^{14}C to fatty acids by liver slices was 2 to 4-fold greater on day 1 and 2 of the cycle than observed in control chicks fed a protein-adequate diet continuously. *In vitro* rates of fatty acid synthesis and malic enzyme activity increased even further when chicks were fed the protein-free diet on the third day of the cycle.

A plot of the influence of dietary protein and fat on lipogenesis in the chick was constructed (Fig. 3). Both dietary protein and fat depress fatty acid synthesis. Interestingly, the influence of dietary protein on hepatic fatty acid synthesis in the chick is greater than that observed when increasing levels of fat were added to the diet. These results suggest that dietary protein and fat depress fatty acid synthesis through different mechanisms.

As discussed in a previous section, fasting or addition of fat to the diet increases plasma-free fatty acid levels, increases hepatic long chain acyl CoA levels, and depresses hepatic fatty acid synthesis. Although addition of protein to the diet markedly depresses hepatic fatty acid synthesis in the chick, plasma-free fatty acid levels are depressed, not increased, as the level of protein in the diet increased

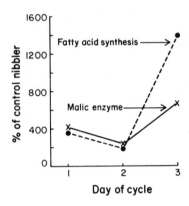

Fig. 2. *Chicks were fed a protein-adequate diet for 2 days and a protein-free diet for the third day of a 3 day cycle. This cycle continued for 21 days. Birds were killed on each day of the 8th cycle. In vitro rates of fatty acid synthesis and malic enzyme activity in livers of these birds were compared with activities observed in control birds fed a protein-adequate diet for the entire experiment. From Leveille and Yeh (1972).*

(Table VIII). To our knowledge, there is only one report in the literature on the influence of dietary protein on hepatic long chain acyl CoA levels in the chick (Yeh and Leveille, 1971). Even though plasma-free fatty acid levels were depressed, hepatic long chain acyl CoA levels were slightly, but significantly, elevated as the level of protein in the diet of the chick was increased from 15% to 35% (Table VIII). It was concluded that factors other than changes in long chain acyl CoA levels were involved in the inhibition of fatty acid synthesis resulting from high protein diets. Possibly a limitation in the availability of cytoplasmic reducing equivalents may have initiated the reduction in hepatic fatty acid synthesis (Yeh and Leveille, 1971).

The redox state of the cell is important in determining the direction of numerous biochemical reactions. Yeh and Leveille (1971) have shown that an increase in dietary pro-

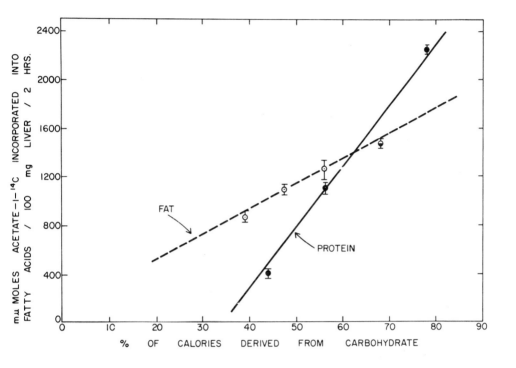

*Fig. 3. Effect of dietary protein and fat level on hepat-
ic lipogenesis in growing chicks. From Yeh and Leveille
(1969).*

tein will increase hepatic gluconeogenesis and thus the need
for reducing equivalents in the chick. An increase in dietary protein depresses the cytoplasmic NADH/NAD$^+$ ratio, as
indicated by the lactate/pyruvate ratio (Table VIII), possibly limiting the availability of reducing equivalents for
fatty acid synthesis. In the rat, at least, changes in the
NADH/NAD$^+$ ratio reflect changes in the NADPH/NADP$^+$ ratio
(Veech *et al.*, 1969). In line with this discussion, we need
to consider that the cytoplasmic NADH/NAD$^+$ ratio is much
higher in the chick than in the rat and further that the
ratio increases when rats are fasted (Krebs, 1967), but de-
dreases when chicks are fasted (Yeh and Leveille, 1967).
The physiological significance of these observations awaits
further study. We also need to note that the chick differs

Table VIII
EFFECT OF DIETARY PROTEIN ON HEPATIC LIPOGENESIS AND
METABOLITE LEVELS IN THE CHICK[a]

	Dietary protein, %	
	15	35
In vivo FAS[b]	9.1 ± 1.3	0.9 ± 0.5
Plasma FFA, μeq/l	793 ± 104	441 ± 15
Hepatic		
Free CoA[c]	93 ± 7	78 ± 8
Acetyl CoA	22 ± 2	20 ± 2
Acyl CoA	21 ± 1	45 ± 2
Lactate	2310 ± 243	1545 ± 124
Pyruvate	39 ± 2	48 ± 6
Lactate/Pyruvate	60 ± 7	33 ± 3

[a]From Yeh and Leveille (1971). Diets fed for 3 weeks.
[b]% of acetate-^{14}C dose recovered in liver fatty acids.
[c]Nanomoles metabolite per gram liver.

from the rat in terms of pathways available for production of NADPH. The pentose pathway, tightly regulated by the NADPH/NADP$^+$ ratio in rat liver (Greenbaum et al., 1971), does not appear to be an important source of NADPH in chick liver (Goodridge, 1968). These observations suggest that the mechanism of involvement of dietary protein in the regulation of lipid metabolism may vary with species.

IV. Dietary Carbohydrate and Meal Pattern

As illustrated in Fig. 3, the quantity of carbohydrate consumed is an important factor in the regulation of lipogenesis; however, the quality of the carbohydrate consumed also needs to be considered. It is well established that dietary fructose stimulates hepatic fatty acid synthesis in the rat to a greater extent than does dietary glucose. We fed fructose and glucose containing diets to rats and chicks to compare the effects of these two carbohydrates in two species known to differ with regard to the major site of fatty acid synthesis. As expected, the activities of fatty acid synthetase, and acetyl CoA carboxylase and the in vitro conversion of acetate-^{14}C to fatty acids by liver slices was elevated in rats fed fructose, rather than glucose containing diets; however, the hepatic lipogenic enzyme activities and in vitro rates of fatty acid synthesis were not changed when fructose replaced glucose as the carbohydrate source in diets of chicks (Table IX). This species-specific response to a dietary stimulus may be related to differences

Table IX
EFFECT OF DIETARY FRUCTOSE ON HEPATIC LIPOGENESIS IN
THE RAT AND CHICK[a]

		Dietary	
	Species	Glucose	Fructose
In vitro FAS	Rat	100	193
	Chick	100	110
Fatty acid synthetase	Rat	100	224
	Chick	100	102
Acetyl CoA carboxylase	Rat	100	182
	Chick	100	117

[a]From Waterman, Romsos and Leveille, unpublished. Diets
fed for 3 weeks. Results expressed as relative values.

in the control of the initial steps of hepatic glycolysis in
rats and chicks. Chick liver does not contain a high K_m
hexokinase similar to glucokinase of rat liver (Ureta *et al.*,
1972, 1973).

In addition to the influence of dietary ingredients on
the control of lipid metabolism, it is now clear that pattern of food intake also alters lipid metabolism. The capacity of adipose tissue preparations from meal-fed rats or
pigs to convert carbohydrate to fatty acids is increased
dramatically (Table X). Thus, it is apparent that factors
which alter food intake pattern may also influence lipid
metabolism.

Table X
INFLUENCE OF PERIODICITY OF EATING ON FATTY ACID SYNTHESIS
AND MALIC ENZYME ACTIVITY IN RAT AND PIG ADIPOSE TISSUE[a]

		Meal pattern	
	Species	Nibbler	Meal fed
In vitro FAS[b]	Rat	663 ± 98	1252 ± 199
	Pig	198 ± 18	551 ± 61
Malic enzyme	Rat	1612 ± 506	3398 ± 811
	Pig	107 ± 9	261 ± 35

[a]From Allee *et al.* (1972); Leveille (1967b). Rats meal
fed one 2 hr. meal per day for 4 weeks. Pigs meal fed one
2 hr. meal every other day for 60 days.
[b]Nanomoles glucose-^{14}C converted to fatty acids per 100 mg
adipose tissue per 2 hr.

V. Dietary Butanediol

1,3-butanediol (BD), a chemically synthesized compound, is converted to β-hydroxybutyrate in the liver. We have studied some of the metabolic effects of BD in rats, pigs, and chicks. Our observations indicate that BD depresses the rate of fatty acid synthesis in rat liver, but not in chick livers, by altering the cellular redox state.

BD, substituted on an equal energy basis for dietary carbohydrate, was fed to rats, pigs, and chicks. Initial studies indicated that substitution of more than 20% of the carbohydrate with BD depressed food intake; consequently, subsequent diets were formulated to contain less than 20% BD energy. Since previous studies reported that addition of BD to diets markedly decreased epididymal fat pad weight and increased liver lipid levels in rats (Mehlman *et al.*, 1966, 1971), we examined the influence of dietary BD on fatty acid synthesis in three species known to differ in the major site of fatty acid synthesis. The *in vitro* rate of glucose-^{14}C conversion to fatty acids in rats, pigs, and chicks fed BD-containing diets is presented in Table XI. Only in rat

Table XI

RATE OF FATTY ACID SYNTHESIS IN RATS, PIGS AND CHICKS
FED DIETS CONTAINING 1,3-BUTANEDIOL[a]

		Butanediol, % of dietary energy	
Species	Tissue	0	17-19
Rat	Liver	100	39
	Adipose	100	83
Pig	Adipose	100	111
Chick	Liver	100	70

[a]From Romsos *et al.* (1974a, 1975b). Diets fed for about 3 weeks. Results expressed as relative values.

liver is the rate of fatty acid synthesis influenced by the addition of BD to the diet. *In vivo* estimates of fatty acid synthesis obtained with glucose-^{14}C and [3]H_2O confirm that dietary BD depressed hepatic lipogenesis, but not adipose tissue lipogenesis, in the rat.

Since addition of BD to the diet influenced hepatic fatty acid synthesis in the rat, but not in the chick, we examined the influence of BD addition directly to the incubation buffer (Table XII). Rat and chick liver slices

Table XII
EFFECT OF 1,3-BUTANEDIOL ADDITION TO THE INCUBATION
BUFFER ON HEPATIC FATTY ACID SYNTHESIS IN THE RAT
AND CHICK[a]

Species	Substrate	Butanediol in buffer	
		0	10 mM
Rat	Glucose	100	46
	Acetate	100	86
Chick	Glucose	100	113
	Acetate	100	117

[a]From Romsos et al. (1974b, 1975b). Results expressed as relative values.

were incubated in the presence or absence of 10 mM BD. BD significantly depressed the rate of glucose, but not of acetate, conversion to fatty acid by rat liver slices. This observation suggested that BD might influence fatty acid synthesis at the level of glucose conversion to acetyl CoA, rather than at the level of acetyl CoA conversion to fatty acids. BD addition to the buffer did not affect glucose conversion to fatty acids in chick liver, in agreement with the influence of dietary BD on hepatic fatty acid synthesis in the chick.

BD is converted to β-hydroxybutyrate in the liver with a concomitant conversion of NAD^+ to NADH (Tate et al., 1971). Since the rate of hepatic glycolysis and the cytoplasmic $NADH/NAD^+$ ratio are inversely related (Gumaa et al., 1971), we postulated that rats fed BD-containing diets might exhibit an increased hepatic $NADH/NAD^+$ ratio, thereby reducing glucose conversion to fatty acids. The lactate/pyruvate ratio, an indicator of the cytoplasmic $NADH/NAD^+$ ratio, was increased when rats were fed BD-containing diets (Table XIII). Unexpectedly, the lactate/pyruvate ratio in chick liver decreased when BD was added to the diet. In addition to the change in the lactate/pyruvate ratio, dietary BD increased hepatic long chain acyl CoA levels in the rat. Hepatic BD metabolism may have spared fatty acid oxidation by altering the mitochondrial redox state. Thus, in the rat, the shift in the cytoplasmic redox state coupled with the increase in the long chain acyl CoA levels may account for the observed depression in the rate of hepatic fatty acid synthesis. It is clear that the chick responds

Table XIII

HEPATIC METABOLITES IN RATS AND CHICKS FED 1,3-BUTANEDIOL[a]

		Butanediol, % of dietary energy	
		0	17-18
Rat	Lactate/Pyruvate ratio	9 ± 1	13 ± 1
	CoA	20 ± 1	21 ± 2
	Acetyl CoA	4 ± 1	5 ± 1
	Acyl CoA	23 ± 1	27 ± 1
Chick	Lactate/Pyruvate ratio	47 ± 6	22 ± 4
	CoA	18 ± 1	22 ± 1
	Acetyl CoA	4 ± 1	5 ± 1
	Acyl CoA	11 ± 1	10 ± 1

[a]From Romsos *et al.* (1974b, 1975b). Results expressed as nanomoles metabolite per gram liver.

differently; the physiological significance of the shift in its cellular redox state following BD ingestion remains to be elucidated.

VI. Conclusions

It is clear that many dietary factors influence lipid metabolism. The inverse relationship between long chain acyl CoA levels coupled with their metabolic effects and rates of fatty acid synthesis in animals fed high fat diets or fasted implicate these metabolites as controllers of fatty acid synthesis. Whether the mechanism whereby polyunsaturated fatty acids exert their effect on lipogenesis, distinct from the effect of saturated fatty acids, involves long chain acyl CoA derivatives remains to be established. Dietary protein appears to influence fatty acid synthesis via a mechanism distinct from the effects of dietary fat; however, further studies are obviously needed to elucidate the mechanism by which dietary protein acts. Species-specific responses to dietary stimuli are apparent and provide an avenue to increase our understanding of the influence of diet on lipid metabolism.

ACKNOWLEDGMENTS

Supported by grant HL-14677 from the National Institutes of Health, U.S. Public Health Service. Journal Article Number 6992. Michigan Agricultural Experiment

Station.

References

Allee, G. L., Baker, D. H., and Leveille, G. A. (1971). *J. Animal Sci.* 33, 1248.

Allee, G. L., Romsos, D. R., Leveille, G. A., and Baker, D. H. (1972). *J. Nutr.* 102, 1115.

Dorsey, J. A., and Porter, J. W. (1968). *J. Biol. Chem.* 243, 3512.

Goodridge, A. G. (1968). *Biochem. J.* 108, 663.

Goodridge, A. G. (1972). *J. Biol. Chem.* 247, 6946.

Greenbaum, A. L., Gumaa, K. A., and McLean, P. (1971). *Arch. Biochem. Biophys.* 143, 617.

Gumaa, K. A., McLean, P., and Greenbaum, A. L. (1971). *Essays in Biochem.* 7, 39.

Halperin, M. L., Robinson, B. H., and Fritz, I. B. (1972). *Proc. Natl. Acad. Sci. U.S.* 69, 1003.

Krebs, H. A. (1967). *Adv. Enz. Reg.* 5, 409.

Leveille, G. A. (1967a). *Proc. Soc. Exp. Biol. Med.* 125, 85.

Leveille, G. A. (1967b). *J. Nutr.* 91, 25.

Leveille, G. A., O'Hea, E. K., and Chakrabarty, K. (1968). *Proc. Soc. Exp. Biol. Med.* 128, 398.

Leveille, G. A., and Yeh, Y. Y. (1972). *J. Nutr.* 102, 733.

Mehlman, M. A., Therriault, D. G., Porter, J. W., Stoewsand, G. A., and Dymsza, H. A. (1966). *J. Nutr.* 88, 215.

Mehlman, M. A., Tobin, R. B., and Johnston, J. B. (1971). *Metabolism* 20, 149.

Musch, K., Ojakiam, M. A., and Williams, M. A. (1974). *Biochim. Biophys. Acta* 337, 343.

O'Hea, E. K., and Leveille, G. A. (1968). *Comp. Biochem. Physiol.* 26, 111.

O'Hea, E. K., and Leveille, G. A. (1969). *J. Nutr.* 99, 388.

O'Hea, E. K., Leveille, G. A., and Sugahara, M. (1970). *Intern. J. Biochem.* 1, 173.

Romsos, D. R., Allee, G. L., and Leveille, G. A. (1971). *Proc. Soc. Exp. Biol. Med.* 137, 570.

Romsos, D. R., Sasse, C., and Leveille, G. A. (1974a). *J. Nutr.* 104, 202.

Romsos, D. R., Belo, P. S., and Leveille, G. A. (1974b). *J. Nutr.* 104, 1438.

Romsos, D. R., Ruiz, S. M., and Leveille, G. A. (1975a). *Comp. Biochem. Physiol.,* in press.

Romsos, D. R., Belo, P. S., Miller, E. R., and Leveille, G. A. (1975b). *J. Nutr.,* in press.

Srere, P. A. (1965). *Biochim. Biophys. Acta* 106, 445.

Tate, R. L., Mehlman, M. A., and Tobin, R. B. (1971). *J. Nutr.* 101, 1719.

Ureta, T., Radojkovic, J., Slebe, J. C., and Reichberg, S. (1972). *Int. J. Biochem.* 3, 103.

Ureta, T., Reichberg, S. B., Radojkovic, J., and Slebe, J. C. (1973). *Comp. Biochem. Physiol.* B45, 445.

Veech, R. L., Eggleston, L. V., and Krebs, H. A. (1969). *Biochem. J.* 115, 609.

Wiley, J. H., and Leveille, G. A. (1973). *J. Nutr.* 103, 829.

Yeh, Y. Y., and Leveille, G. A. (1969). *J. Nutr.* 98, 356.

Yeh, Y. Y., and Leveille, G. A. (1971). *J. Nutr.* 101, 911.

Yeh, Y. Y., Leveille, G. A., and Wiley, J. H. (1970). *J. Nutr.* 100, 917.

Effect of (-)-Hydroxycitrate on
Lipid Metabolism

ANN C. SULLIVAN

I. Introduction

The major homeostatic function of fatty acid synthesis
is the conversion of carbohydrate and its metabolites into
lipid during periods of excessive intake relative to immediate energy demand. The fatty acids are converted to
triglycerides, transported in the blood as lipoprotein complexes and stored in the adipose tissue. Obesity and hyperlipidemia are diseases characterized by an excessive accumulation of lipid in the adipose tissue and blood, respectively. An agent capable of reducing the conversion of
carbohydrate and its metabolites into lipid, e.g., by inhibiting fatty acid synthesis, may be therapeutically useful in these diseases.

(-)-Hydroxycitrate was reported to be a potent competitive inhibitor of ATP citrate lyase (K_i 0.2 µM to 0.6 µM)
by Watson et al. (1969). This enzyme catalyzes the extramitochondrial cleavage of citrate to acetyl CoA and oxaloacetate. If ATP citrate lyase is an important enzyme in
maintaining the acetyl CoA pool in vivo, then inhibition of
this enzyme should reduce this pool thus limiting the availability of 2-carbon units for fatty acid and cholesterol
synthesis.

In assessing the effects of (-)-hydroxycitrate on lipid
metabolism, an understanding of its potential interaction
with other enzymes and pathways is important. (-)-Hydroxy-
citrate was shown to be a competitive inhibitor of mitochondrial aconitase (Sullivan, 1973; Cheema-Dhadli et al.,
1973), citrate synthase (Glusker and Srere, 1973; Cheema-
Dhadli et al., 1973), and $NADP^+$-linked isocitrate dehydrogenase (Cheema-Dhadli et al., 1973). These data suggested
that if (-)-hydroxycitrate were transported into the

mitochondria, then respiration and energy production could be significantly affected. However, Cheema-Dhadli *et al.* (1973) demonstrated that (-)-hydroxycitrate was a very weak substrate for the mitochondrial tricarboxylate carrier, being transported at only 2% to 9% of the rate observed with citrate. Other observations supported this finding. Using a reconstituted cell-free system from rat liver consisting of mitochondria and particle-free cytoplasm, Watson and Lowenstein (1970) observed that (-)-hydroxycitrate inhibited fatty acid synthesis, but had no effect on respiration, phosphorylation or citrate accumulation. (-)-Hydroxycitrate did not alter $^{14}CO_2$ production in isolated hepatocytes even at concentrations which maximally inhibited fatty acid and cholesterol synthesis (Sullivan *et al.*, 1974d). Similar results were reported by Goodridge (1973). The production of ATP (Decker and Barth, 1973) and ketone bodies (Decker and Barth, 1973; Brunengraber and Lowenstein, 1973) was unchanged when rat livers were perfused with (-)-hydroxycitrate. These studies demonstrated that the extent of transport of (-)-hydroxycitrate into the mitochondria was insufficient to alter a number of mitochondrial functions.

The following summarizes our present understanding of how (-)-hydroxycitrate affects lipid metabolism.

II. Stereoisomers of Hydroxycitrate

A. OCCURRENCE AND ISOLATION

Von Lippman (1883) first described the occurrence of hydroxycitrate as a minor component of sugar beets. Martius and Maue (1941) synthesized hydroxycitrate from *trans*-aconitic acid and resolved the four stereoisomers. (-)-Hydroxycitrate was isolated by Lewis *et al.* (1964) and Lewis and Neelakantan (1965) as the γ-lactone from the dried fruit rinds of *Garcinia cambogia* where its concentration approached 20 to 30%. These dried rinds from *Garcinia cambogia* (also called "Malabar Tamarind") are utilized for culinary purposes in India and commercially in a fish preservation process (Lewis and Neelakantan, 1965). Griebel (1939, 1942) prepared (+)-*allo*-hydroxycitrate from the calyxes of *Hisbiscus sabdariffa*. The isolation and properties of these two naturally occurring isomers of hydroxycitrate have been described recently (Lewis, 1969). The absolute configuration of the lactones of (-)-hydroxycitrate and (+)-*allo*-hydroxycitrate have been determined by X-ray

crystallography by Glusker *et al*. (1969, 1971) and by NMR
infrared studies by Boll *et al*. (1969).

B. NOMENCLATURE

Confusion has arisen regarding the nomenclature used
for identifying the stereoisomers of hydroxycitrate. Lewis
(1969) designated (±)-hydroxycitrate as *erythro* and (±)-
allo-hydroxycitrate as *threo*. However, these designations
are opposite to the *erythro* and *threo* nomenclature as defined by Cram (1952) and Cahn *et al*. (1956) and used by
Horikawa and Masuyama (1965). To avoid these and other
confusions, Srere (1972) proposed that the derivatives of
citrate retain the original numbering and stereochemistry
of the parent citrate molecule. This "parent numbering"
system indicated by the prefix (*pn* cit) was developed and
described by Glusker and Srere (1973). The usefulness of
this system becomes obvious when, for example, the hydroxycitrates and fluorocitrates are being compared in the same
experimental system.

ATP citrate lyase has the same stereospecificity as
citrate synthase (Spencer and Lowenstein, 1962; Bhaduri and
Srere, 1963). Carbons 4 and 5 of citrate are derived from
acetyl CoA in the citrate synthase reaction and these are
the same stereochemically as the carbon atoms which become
acetyl CoA during the cleavage of citrate catalyzed by ATP
citrate lyase. The absolute configuration of the stereoisomers of hydroxycitrate according to the Fischer convention are illustrated in Fig. 1. Note that (-)-hydroxy-
citrate and (-)-*allo*-hydroxycitrate have the hydroxyl group
(bold face type) on the acetyl CoA-derived portion of the
molecule, whereas the hydroxyl group of (+)-hydroxycitrate
and (+)-*allo*-hydroxycitrate is on the oxaloacetate-derived
portion.

III. Effects on Lipid Biosynthesis

A. PRECURSORS OF ACETYL CoA FOR LIPID SYNTHESIS

Since (-)-hydroxycitrate is a competitive inhibitor of
ATP citrate lyase, its effectiveness as an inhibitor of
lipid biosynthesis depends on the extent of the contribution
of ATP citrate lyase to the extramitochondrial acetyl CoA
pool. During periods of excessive carbohydrate intake

145

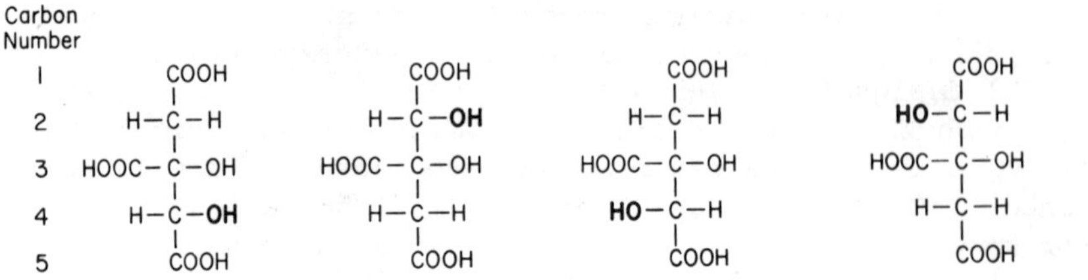

Carbon
Number

1	COOH	COOH	COOH	COOH
2	H—C—H	H—C—**OH**	H—C—H	**HO**—C—H
3	HOOC—C—OH	HOOC—C—OH	HOOC—C—OH	HOOC—C—OH
4	H—C—**OH**	H—C—H	**HO**—C—H	H—C—H
5	COOH	COOH	COOH	COOH

(−)-Hydroxycitrate   (+)-Hydroxycitrate   (−)-*Allo*-hydroxycitrate   (+)-*Allo*-hydroxycitrate

(pn_{cit})-(4S)-4− (pn_{cit})-(2R)-2− (pn_{cit})-(4R)-4− (pn_{cit})-(2S)-2−

Fig. 1. *Absolute configuration of the stereoisomers of hydroxycitrate according to the Fischer convention. The hydroxyl group which is unique to each stereoisomer is shown in bold face type. The designations of the stereoisomers in the parent numbering system* (pn_{cit}) *of Glusker and Srere (1973) are indicated.*

relative to immediate energy requirements, the surplus acetyl CoA produced, by the oxidation of pyruvate in the mitochondria must be transferred to the cytoplasm for conversion to fatty acids. Direct translocation of the thioester is impossible since the mitochondrial membrane is impermeable to acetyl CoA (Lardy, 1966). Three mechanisms have been postulated for the translocation of acetyl CoA as indicated in Fig. 2: (1) as acetate followed by reactivation to acetyl CoA in the cytosol by acetyl CoA synthetase (Kornacker and Lowenstein, 1965; Barth et al., 1971, 1972b); (2) as acetyl carnitine through the action of acetyl carnitine transferase (Fritz and Yue, 1964); and (3) as citrate with subsequent cleavage to acetyl CoA and oxaloacetate by ATP citrate lyase (Srere and Bhaduri, 1962; Spencer and Lowenstein, 1962; Bhaduri and Srere, 1963; Inoue et al., 1966; Lowenstein, 1968; Daikuhara et al., 1968). Citrate is generally accepted as the primary cytoplasmic precursor of acetyl CoA in nonruminant mammals. Citrate could be transported to the cytoplasm directly or indirectly through the intermediate formation of glutamate as suggested by D'Adamo and Haft (1965). However, this possible transport of the acetyl group as glutamate has recently been

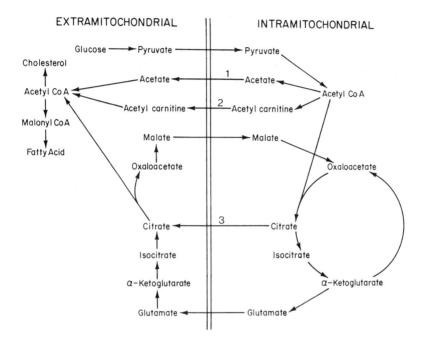

EXTRAMITOCHONDRIAL   **INTRAMITOCHONDRIAL**

Fig. 2. *Carbon flux during the conversion of carbohydrate and its metabolites into lipid. Three mechanisms which have been postulated for the translocation of acetyl CoA from the mitochondrion to the cytoplasm are illustrated: 1) as acetate followed by reactivation to acetyl CoA by acetyl CoA synthetase, 2) as acetyl carnitine through the action of acetyl carnitine transferase, and 3) as citrate with subsequent cleavage to acetyl CoA and oxaloacetate by ATP citrate lyase.*

questioned (Lowenstein, 1970).

Most of the studies supporting this key role of citrate in the production of extramitochondrial acetyl CoA were performed in rat liver. However, the importance of the ATP citrate lyase pathway in the production of acetyl CoA in mouse liver has been questioned by Rous (1971, 1973, 1974). Recently, the physiological significance of acetate as a citrate-independent precursor has been reemphasized (Barth *et al.*, 1971, 1972b).

B. COMPARISON OF THE STEREOISOMERS OF HYDROXYCITRATE

The stereospecific requirements of the inhibition of ATP citrate lyase by (-)-hydroxycitrate were investigated by comparing the effects of the 4 stereoisomers on fatty acid biosynthesis (Sullivan et al., 1972). When the isomers were studied in an in vitro rat liver system which measure the incorporation of $(1,5 ^{14}-C)$ citrate into fatty acids, several differences were apparent: 1) only (-)-hydroxycitrate markedly reduced lipogenesis, 2) (-)-allo-hydroxycitrate demonstrated weak inhibitory activity, and 3) higher concentrations of (+)-hydroxycitrate stimulated fatty acid synthesis (Table I).

Table I

EFFECT OF (-)-HYDROXYCITRATE AND ITS STEREOISOMERS ON IN VITRO LIPOGENESIS[a]

Treatment	Concentration	Rate of Lipogenesis[b]			
		5 mM Citrate[c]	Per Cent of Control	10 mM Citrate[c]	Per Cent of Control
	mM	mμmoles converted[b]	%	mμmoles converted[b]	%
Control		1381 ± 39		2321 ± 91	
(-)-Hydroxycitrate	1.0	388 ± 26 **	28	1067 ± 62 **	46
	0.1	665 ± 34 **	48	1496 ± 232 **	65
(+)-Hydroxycitrate	1.0	2145 ± 202 **	155	3032 ± 239 **	131
	0.1	1432 ± 144	104	2099 ± 306	90
(-)-Allo-hydroxycitrate	1.0	1107 ± 117 *	80	2041 ± 285	88
	0.1	1298 ± 158	94	2264 ± 177	98
(+)-Allo-hydroxycitrate	1.0	1814 ± 88 **	131	2500 ± 377	108
	0.1	1431 ± 82	104	2388 ± 360	103

[a] Reproduced from Sullivan et al. (1972) by kind permission of the Cambridge University Press.

[b] Five rats were prefasted 48 hours, then meal-fed the G-70 diet for 13 days. High speed supernatants of liver (105,000 x g for 30 min) were pooled and assayed for 20 min at $37°$ in 5 mM citrate or 10 mM citrate and the stereoisomers of (—)-hydroxycitrate at the concentrations indicated.

[c] Data are expressed as nmoles [^{14}C]citrate converted into lipid per g liver per 30 min. Data may be converted into [^{14}C]citrate converted into lipid per mg protein by dividing by 20. Each value is the mean ± SE of results from 4 assays for all hydroxycitrate groups and 7 assays for the control group.

* $p < 0.05$

** $p < 0.01$

To examine the ability of these isomers to influence lipogenesis in vivo, a model system was developed to determine in vivo rates of lipid biosynthesis. In this system, rats were induced to synthesize lipid at an elevated rate under conditions which included meal-feeding a high carbohydrate diet (G-70 diet), etc. (Sullivan et al., 1971).

As described in Table II, the oral administration of only (-)-hydroxycitrate reduced significantly the *in vivo* rate of hepatic lipogenesis as measured by the conversion of (^{14}C) alanine into fatty acids. The other isomers were ineffective in significantly altering fatty acid synthesis under these conditions. In other experiments, a significant depression of lipogenesis by (-)-hydroxycitrate was demonstrated using ^3H_2O, (^{14}C) lactate and (^{14}C) glucose as precursors.

Table II

Effect of (-)-Hydroxycitrate Lactone and its Stereoisomers on

In Vivo Lipogenesis[a]

Treatment[b]	Number of rats	Rate of lipogenesis	
		nmoles [^{14}C]alanine converted[c]	Per cent of control %
Control	21	1022 ± 58	
(-)-Hydroxycitrate	39	589 ± 52 **	58
(+)-Hydroxycitrate	5	1189 ± 308	116
(-)-Allo-hydroxycitrate	5	1001 ± 108	98
(+)-Allo-hydroxycitrate	5	1059 ± 190	104

[a] Reproduced from Sullivan et al. (1972) by kind permission of the Cambridge University Press.

[b] Rats were prefasted 48 hours, then meal-fed the G-70 diet for 12 days. On day 13 the rats were administered saline or the stereoisomers (2.63 mmoles/kg) by stomach tube 60 min before feeding and the livers were assayed immediately after the 3-hour feeding period.

[c] Data are expressed as nmoles [^{14}C]alanine converted into lipid per g liver per 30 min. Each value is the group mean ± SE.

** $p < 0.01$

C. ACUTE ADMINISTRATION OF (-)-HYDROXYCITRATE

The observation that (-)-hydroxycitrate inhibited significantly hepatic fatty acid synthesis *in vivo* raised several interesting points regarding its effect on: 1) cholesterol, triglyceride, and phospholipid biosynthesis in liver, 2) lipid synthesis in other tissues, and 3) the extent and duration of the inhibition of lipogenesis. The following summarizes these key points which have been discussed in detail (Sullivan *et al.*, 1972, 1974a).

1) (-)-Hydroxycitrate depressed the synthesis of all lipid classes including cholesterol, cholesterol esters,

triglycerides, diglycerides, and phospholipids. There was an equivalent inhibition of the incorporation of ^3H_2O and (^{14}C) alanine into the various lipid classes when isolated hepatocytes were incubated in the presence of (-)-hydroxy-citrate. Although the extent of synthesis of the various lipids was significantly reduced with (-)-hydroxycitrate, the distribution of lipids synthesized in the hepatocytes in the presence or absence of (-)-hydroxycitrate was essential-ly identical as described in Table III. Table IV demon-strates that the *in vivo* hepatic synthesis of fatty acids

Table III

EFFECT OF 2 mM (—)-HYDROXYCITRATE ON THE DISTRIBUTION OF LIPIDS
BIOSYNTHESIZED IN ISOLATED LIVER CELLS[a, b]

LIPID CLASS	CONTROL		(—)-HYDROXYCITRATE	
	% OF TOTAL	% OF PHOSPHO-LIPID TOTAL	% OF TOTAL	% OF PHOSPHO-LIPID TOTAL
CHOLESTEROL ESTERS	2.1 ± 0.3		1.6 ± 0.2	
TRIGLYCERIDES	47.0 ± 1.1		52.0 ± 0.6**	
CHOLESTEROL	11.1 ± 0.3		9.6 ± 0.3**	
FREE FATTY ACIDS	1.1 ± 0.1		1.2 ± 0.2	
DIGLYCERIDES	7.1 ± 0.5		5.9 ± 0.2*	
PHOSPHOLIPIDS	29.7 ± 0.8		28.5 ± 0.3	
PHOSPHATIDYL ETHANOLAMINE		7.4 ± 0.4		7.1 ± 0.2
PHOSPHATIDYL CHOLINE		19.4 ± 0.7		17.6 ± 0.3
POLAR		1.9 ± 0.1		2.2 ± 0.2

[a]Rates of total lipid biosynthesized in control flasks were 2.55 ± 0.09 nmoles [^{14}C]alanine converted/mg dry wt/60 min and 113.04 ± 8.34 nmoles ^3H_2O converted/mg dry wt/60 min. The corresponding rates in (—)-hydroxycitrate flasks were 1.41 ± 0.03 nmoles [^{14}C]alanine converted/mg dry wt/60 min and 82.59 ± 3.42 nmoles ^3H_2O converted/mg dry wt/60 min. (—)Hydroxy-citrate rates were significantly less than control ($p < 0.001$) Data are expressed as the mean % of total ± SE.

[b]The lipid classes were separated by thin layer chromatography using glass fiber paper and then counted.

*$p < 0.05$ **$p < 0.01$

and cholesterol as measured by the incorporation of (^{14}C) alanine was significantly reduced in a dose-dependent man-ner after the oral administration of (-)-hydroxycitrate. An equivalent inhibition of the synthesis of both types of lipid was observed. Similar results were obtained using ^3H_2O and (^{14}C) glucose as precursors. (-)-Hydroxycitrate did not affect the mitochondrial production of acetyl CoA (see Introduction), but did inhibit lipogenesis and cho-lesterogenesis to a similar extent. These data supported

Table IV

Inhibition of In Vivo Fatty Acid and Cholesterol Synthesis after
Oral Administration of (-)-Hydroxycitrate Lactone [a]

Treatment [b]	Number of rats	Dose mmoles/kg	Fatty Acids		Cholesterol	
			nmoles [^{14}C]alanine converted [c]	Inhibition %	nmoles [^{14}C]alanine converted [c]	Inhibition %
Saline	5		1552 ± 153		27.8 ± 3.9	
(-)-Hydroxycitrate	5	5.26	303 ± 22 **	80	8.6 ± 1.5 **	69
(-)-Hydroxycitrate	5	3.95	449 ± 108 **	71	16.7 ± 2.0 **	40
(-)-Hydroxycitrate	5	2.63	500 ± 155 **	68	18.1 ± 5.5 **	35
(-)-Hydroxycitrate	5	1.32	1046 ± 141	33	31.0 ± 4.5	0
(-)-Hydroxycitrate	5	0.66	1200 ± 175	23	30.0 ± 7.2	0

[a] Reproduced from Sullivan et al. (1972) by kind permission of the Cambridge University Press.

[b] Rats were prefasted 48 hours, then meal-fed the G-70 diet for 7 days. On day 8 the rats were administered either saline or (—)-hydroxycitrate lactone by stomach tube 60 min before feeding and the livers were asayed immediately after the 3-hour feeding period.

[c] Data are expressed as nmoles ^{14}C-alanine converted into fatty acids or cholesterol per g liver per 30 min. Each value is the group mean ± S.E.

** $p < 0.01$

the concept that a common cytoplasmic acetyl CoA pool was utilized for fatty acid and cholesterol synthesis, and, therefore, the conversion of acetyl CoA to HMG CoA in cholesterogenesis was a cytoplasmic rather than mitochondrial process.

Several other investigators have reported that (-)-hydroxycitrate depressed fatty acid and cholesterol synthesis. Lowenstein (1971) demonstrated that the intraperitoneal administration of (-)-hydroxycitrate reduced significantly the *in vivo* incorporation of ^3H_2O into fatty acids in rat liver. Barth *et al.* (1972a) and Brunengraber *et al.* (1972) reported an inhibition of cholesterol synthesis when rat livers were perfused with (-)-hydroxycitrate. In human epidermis (Ziboh, unpublished observations) and guinea pig ear skin (Wheatley *et al.*, 1973), (-)-hydroxycitrate suppressed the incorporation of (^{14}C) glucose into fatty acids and cholesterol.

2) The oral administration of (-)-hydroxycitrate inhibited significantly the *in vivo* rates of lipogenesis in

151

several tissues known to convert carbohydrate into fatty acids, namely, liver, adipose tissue, and small intestine. Although the rates at which (^{14}C) alanine was converted into fatty acids by the 3 tissues differed markedly (adipose tissue > liver > small intestine), all were depressed significantly in a dose-dependent manner by (-)-hydroxycitrate (Sullivan et al., 1974a).

3) The extent and duration of the inhibition of fatty acid synthesis produced by (-)-hydroxycitrate was an interesting problem. To answer this question, in vivo rates of hepatic lipogenesis, as determined by the conversion of (^{14}C) alanine and ^3H_2O into fatty acids, were examined over a 24 hour period. Figure 3 illustrates that a single oral dose of (-)-hydroxycitrate administered to rats given the same amount of food as controls depressed hepatic lipogenesis for the 8 hour period following the initiation of the meal when control animals demonstrated elevated rates of synthesis. The possibility that at later times a "frame shift" in lipogenic rates would occur in treated animals, i.e., that the carbons and electrons diverted from hepatic fatty acid synthesis during this 8 hour period after feeding would be incorporated into lipid at later intervals was not substantiated. The slightly increased rates observed from 8 hours to 24 hours in the (-)-hydroxycitrate treated animals compared to controls were not significant.

The extent of the diversion of carbohydrate and its metabolites from lipid synthesis by (-)-hydroxycitrate was considerable. The metabolic fate of these diverted carbons and electrons has been the subject of intensive investigation in our laboratory. The most marked change in metabolic flux that we have observed after (-)-hydroxycitrate treatment during the 8 hour period when fatty acid synthesis was maximally reduced was a significant increase in the rate of hepatic glycogenesis. This increased rate paralleled a significantly greater deposition of glycogen (approximately 20%) in (-)-hydroxycitrate treated rats (Sullivan et al., 1974c). We have detected no significant changes in the following in vivo parameters after the oral administration of (-)-hydroxycitrate: 1) oxidation of carbohydrate, 2) blood glucose levels, 3) serum insulin levels, and 4) urinary glucose levels (Sullivan et al., unpublished observations). As discussed in the Introduction, (-)-hydroxycitrate had no effect on a number of mitochondrial systems, including respiration, citrate accumulation (Watson and Lowenstein, 1970), phosphorylation (Watson and Lowenstein,

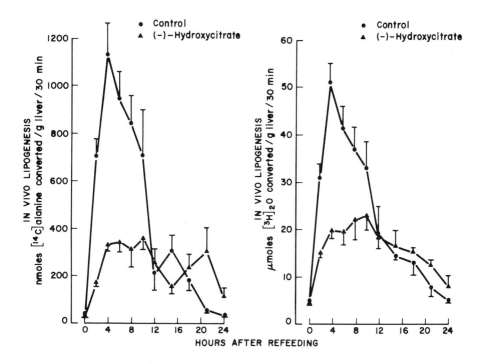

*Fig. 3. Effect of the oral administration of (-)-hydroxy-
citrate on the in vivo rate of hepatic lipogenesis determined over a 24 hour period. Rats were prefasted 48 hours,
then meal-fed the G-70 diet for 6 days. On day 7, 55 rats
each were given orally either saline or (-)-hydroxycitrate
(2.63 mmoles/kg) directly before receiving 8.7 g of food.
The in vivo rate of lipogenesis was determined using the
(^{14}C) alanine and $^{3}H_2O$ pulse at the indicated times. The
vertical bar gives the SE of the mean (5 rats per point).
Nmoles (^{14}C) alanine and μmoles $^{3}H_2O$ converted into lipid
in the (-)-hydroxycitrate treated animals were significantly
different from controls at hour 2, 4, 6, and 8 (p < 0.05).
From Sullivan et al. (1974a). Reprinted by courtesy of the
American Oil Chemists' Society.*

1970; Decker and Barth, 1973), and ketone body production
(Decker and Barth, 1973; Brunengraber and Lowenstein, 1973).

D. ACTIVATION OF ACETYL CoA CARBOXYLASE BY (-)-HYDROXY-
CITRATE

Acetyl CoA carboxylase from mammalian sources was activated by various carboxylic acids (Martin and Vagelos, 1962;
Waite and Wakil, 1962; Vagelos et al., 1963) of which
citrate and isocitrate were the most effective (Matsuhashi
et al., 1964). Electron microscopic studies demonstrated
that the active configuration of this enzyme consisted of a
polymeric filamentous structure which was both easily dis-
sociated into protomeric units and readily reconstituted by
citrate, isocitrate, and carboxylic acids. Thus, the level
of activity of acetyl CoA carboxylase appeared to be controlled by tricarboxylic acids, although critical proof of
this in vivo has been difficult to obtain.

Hackenschmidt et al. (1972) and Cheema-Dhadli et al.
(1973) demonstrated that (-)-hydroxycitrate stimulated the
activity of acetyl CoA carboxylase. A kinetic analysis
proved that (-)-hydroxycitrate was an effector of the V_{max}
type (Hackenschmidt et al., 1972) in contrast to citrate
which produced an activation of the K_m type (Hashimoto and
Numa, 1971). As discussed previously, Barth et al. (1972a)
and Decker and Barth (1973) demonstrated in the perfused
rat liver system that (-)-hydroxycitrate inhibited the incorporation of ^3H_2O into fatty acids and cholesterol. They
also reported that if 10 mM (1-^{14}C) acetate were added to
the perfusion medium containing ^3H_2O and 1.1 mM (-)-hydroxy-
citrate, then the incorporation of ^{14}C and ^3H was stimulated
into fatty acids and inhibited into cholesterol. (A careful
examination of these results suggests that these effects
were not statistically significant.) Since the addition of
acetate alone did not affect fatty acid or cholesterol
synthesis, the authors interpreted their data as follows:
1) in the absence of added acetate, (-)-hydroxycitrate inhibited the incorporation of ^3H_2O into fatty acids and
cholesterol because it reduced the production of acetyl CoA,
2) in the presence of acetate, (-)-hydroxycitrate stimulated
fatty acid synthesis from (^{14}C) acetate and ^3H_2O because it
activated acetyl CoA carboxylase, and 3) (-)-hydroxycitrate
inhibited cholesterol synthesis from (^{14}C) acetate and ^3H_2O
because the concomitant stimulation of fatty acid synthesis
depleted the acetyl CoA pool thus limiting the availability
of 2-carbon precursors for sterol production.

We have independently examined the interrelationships
between (-)-hydroxycitrate and exogenous acetate on hepatic

fatty acid and cholesterol synthesis in fed and fasted rats. Our results indicate the problems that can arise from interpreting metabolic flux data in the nutritionally undefined perfused liver system used by Barth *et al.* (1972a) and Decker and Barth (1973). In our experiments, the *in vivo* rates of fatty acid and cholesterol synthesis were measured in fed and fasted rats which were divided into 3 groups according to the type of radioactive precursor administered. Rats received either: a) (^{14}C) alanine and ^3H_2O, b) ($2-^{14}C$) acetate and ^3H_2O or c) (^{14}C) alanine and (^3H) acetate.

The administration of (-)-hydroxycitrate to the fed rat significantly reduced the incorporation of (^{14}C) alanine and ^3H_2O into fatty acids (Fig. 4). Although the conversion of either (^{14}C) acetate or (^3H) acetate was significantly increased, this did not reflect a real stimulation of fatty acid synthesis since the incorporation of ^3H_2O was significantly inhibited. Since (-)-hydroxycitrate reduced the acetyl CoA pool in the fed rat, the increased incorporation of labeled acetate into fatty acids reflected a decreased dilution of the radiolabel by the endogenous pool. Thus, (-)-hydroxycitrate did not produce a significant stimulation of fatty acid synthesis via activation of acetyl CoA carboxylase *in vivo* in the fed animal, probably because the endogenous citrate levels were sufficiently high to accomplish this function. This interpretation of our data was reinforced by the similarity of the effect of (-)-hydroxycitrate in the fed rat on cholesterogenesis (Fig. 5) and lipogenesis. Acetyl CoA carboxylase is involved in the synthesis of fatty acids, but does not catalyze any reactions involved in sterol biosynthesis. Therefore, any effect on this enzyme produced by (-)-hydroxycitrate should give different results in these *in vivo* labeling studies on fatty acid and cholesterol synthesis. However, a comparison of the data in Fig. 4 (fatty acid synthesis) and Fig. 5 (cholesterol synthesis) demonstrated identical trends in labeling patterns with and without (-)-hydroxycitrate administration.

An interesting observation was made when these same experiments were conducted in the fasted rat. (-)-Hydroxycitrate stimulated significantly the *in vivo* rate of fatty acid synthesis as measured by ^3H_2O incorporation, proving that the concomitant increases observed in (^{14}C) acetate and (^3H) acetate conversion were real (Fig. 6). These data suggested that: 1) (-)-hydroxycitrate activated acetyl CoA carboxylase *in vivo* in the fasted rat and 2) the activation of acetyl CoA carboxylase by tricarboxylic acids does

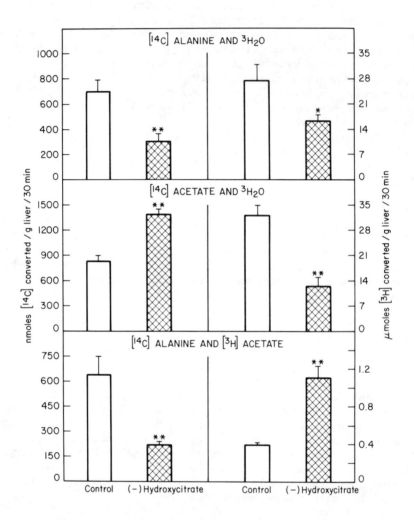

Fig. 4. Influence of (-)-hydroxycitrate on fatty acid synthesis from several precursors in the fed rat. Six groups of 9 to 10 rats each were prefasted 48 hours, then meal-fed the G-70 diet for 6 to 9 days. They were then administered saline or (-)-hydroxycitrate by stomach tube directly before the meal. Livers were assayed for in vivo rates of fatty acid synthesis immediately after the 3 hour feeding Fig. 4 legend continued on next page.

occur *in vivo* and has physiological significance. The demonstration of activation of the acetyl CoA carboxylase by (-)-hydroxycitrate in the fasted rat was possible due to the significantly decreased citrate levels present during fasting, which were described by Start and Newsholme (1971). (^{14}C) Alanine conversion to fatty acids in the fasted rat was unchanged by (-)-hydroxycitrate administration, suggesting that carbon flux into fatty acids in the fasted rat did not involve ATP citrate lyase, i.e., the production of acetyl CoA did not depend upon the cleavage of citrate.

In contrast to fatty acid synthesis, (-)-hydroxycitrate did not alter the *in vivo* rates of cholesterogenesis from (^{14}C) alanine and ^3H_2O in the fasted rat (Fig. 7). These data were expected since acetyl CoA carboxylase did not catalyze any reactions involved in cholesterogenesis. The significant increase in the incorporation of (^{14}C) acetate and (^{3}H) acetate into cholesterol in the fasted rat given (-)-hydroxycitrate is unexplained at the present time.

These experiments further demonstrated the preferential usefulness of ^3H_2O for the measurement of rates of lipid biosynthesis. ^3H_2O is not subject to alterations in pool size which may change the specific activity of ^{14}C precursors, e.g., the pool dilution effects observed with (^{14}C) and (^{3}H) acetate in Fig. 4. The use of ^3H_2O provides a measure of the total rate of fatty acid and cholesterol synthesis independent of source of carbon precursors for acetyl CoA (Jungas, 1968; Lowenstein, 1967; Brunengraber *et al.*, 1972).

Fig. 4 continued. period. Radiolabeled precursors were given intravenously 30 minutes before sacrifice. They consisted of the following made to a final volume of 0.25 ml with saline: 1) 12.3 mg alanine, 5 μCi (^{14}C) alanine, 30.6 mg α-ketoglutarate (as an amine acceptor for transaminase) and 1 mCi ^3H_2O, 2) 15 mg acetate, 15 μCi (2-^{14}C) acetate and 1 mCi ^3H_2O, and 3) 12.3 mg alanine, 5 μCi (^{14}C) alanine, 30.6 mg α-ketoglutarate, 15 mg acetate and 15 μCi (^{3}H) acetate. Data are expressed as nmoles (^{14}C) alanine, nmoles (^{14}C) acetate, μmoles ^3H_2O or μmoles (^{3}H) acetate converted into fatty acids per g liver per 30 minutes. The vertical bar gives the SE of the mean. *p < 0.05. **p < 0.01.

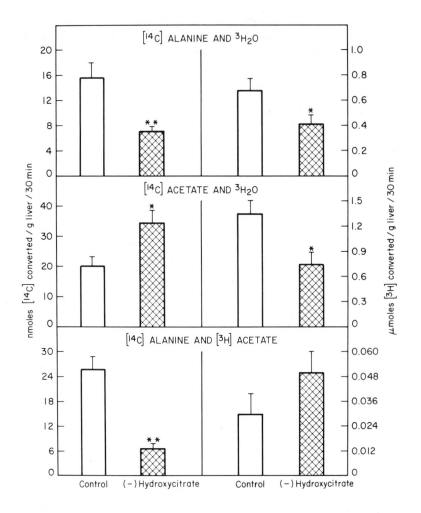

Fig. 5.   Influence of (-)-hydroxycitrate on cholesterol synthesis from several precursors in the fed rat.   Six groups
of 9 to 10 rats each were prefasted 48 hours, then meal-fed
the G-70 diet for 6 to 9 days.   They were then administered
saline or (-)-hydroxycitrate by stomach tube directly before the meal.   Livers were assayed for in vivo rates of
cholesterol synthesis immediately after the 3 hour feeding
Fig. 5 legend continued on next page.

E. CHRONIC ADMINISTRATION OF (-)-HYDROXYCITRATE

The effects of the chronic administration of (-)-hydroxycitrate on hepatic lipogenesis were compared to those observed after a single dose. Fig. 8 demonstrates the *in vitro* rate of fatty acid synthesis in rats administered varying concentrations of (-)-hydroxycitrate orally for 30 days. The upper curve illustrates the observed *in vitro* rate and the lower curve presents the lipogenic rate when 1 mM (-)-hydroxycitrate was added to each assay. A similar level of significant inhibition was observed regardless of the control *in vitro* lipogenic rate. However, the unexpected finding was the significant increase (1.5 to 2.1-fold) in the *in vitro* rate of hepatic lipogenesis in animals receiving 2.63, 1.32, and 0.66 mmoles/kg of (-)-hydroxycitrate for 30 days. Since the *in vitro* assay provided a measure of the activities of ATP citrate lyase, acetyl CoA carboxylase and fatty acid synthetase, the observed rate increases suggested that the lipogenic enzyme levels and/or activities were elevated as a result of a prolonged period of daily suppression of fatty acid synthesis by (-)-hydroxycitrate. The extent and duration of the inhibition of *in vivo* lipogenesis produced by (-)-hydroxycitrate was identical regardless of the number of days of administration. The dose-dependent inhibition of *in vivo* lipogenesis after 30 days of (-)-hydroxycitrate administration illustrated in Fig. 9 was similar to that observed after acute administration (Table III). It was expected that the rates determined from ^3H_2O were less depressed than the rates from (^{14}C) alanine, since ^3H_2O provided a measure of the total rate of lipid synthesis independent of the carbon precursors for acetyl CoA.

Fig. 5 continued. period. Radiolabeled precursors were given intravenously 30 minutes before sacrifice as described in the legend of Fig. 4. Data are expressed as nmoles (^{14}C) alanine, nmoles (^{14}C) acetate, μmoles ^3H_2O or μmoles (^3H) acetate converted into cholesterol per g liver per 30 minutes. The vertical bar gives the SE of the mean. *p < 0.05. **p < 0.01.

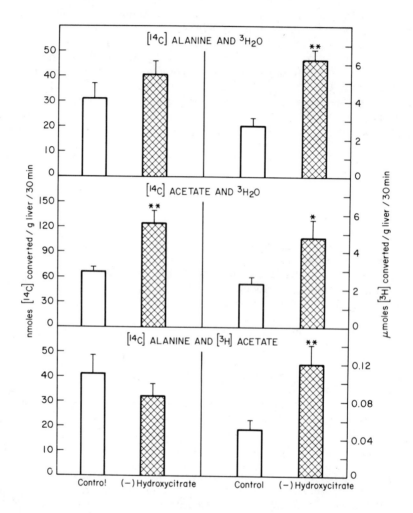

Fig. 6. Influence of (-)-hydroxycitrate on fatty acid synthesis from several precursors in the fasted rat. Six groups of 9 to 10 rats each were prefasted 48 hours, then meal-fed the G-70 diet for 6 to 9 days. They were then administered saline or (-)-hydroxycitrate by stomach tube 21 hours after the last meal. Livers were assayed for in vivo rates of fatty acid synthesis 3 hours later. Radio-labeled precursors were given intravenously 30 minutes
Fig. 6 legend continued on next page.

IV. Effects of (-)-Hydroxycitrate on Lipid Accumulation

A. SERUM TRIGLYCERIDE LEVELS

To investigate the effect of (-)-hydroxycitrate on blood lipid levels, several model systems were utilized. A hypertriglyceridemic rat model was employed using fructose as the stimulus. When either fed or fasted rats received 10% fructose in the drinking water for a 28 hour period, their serum triglyceride levels approximately doubled (Fig. 10). If (-)-hydroxycitrate was administered orally at 3 intervals during the time of fructose availability, the elevated triglyceride levels were significantly reduced regardless of the nutritional status of the rat, i.e., fed or fasted. Fig. 11 demonstrates that a significantly increased *in vivo* rate of hepatic lipogenesis was one mechanism causing the hypertriglyceridemia produced by fructose. This elevation in fatty acid synthesis was particularly marked in the fasted rats receiving fructose. (-)-Hydroxycitrate administration inhibited significantly these fructose-induced elevated rates of *in vivo* fatty acid synthesis in both fed and fasted animals. Similar results were obtained when (-)-hydroxycitrate was given to rats meal-fed a high fructose diet.

Our preliminary investigations have demonstrated that the oral administration of (-)-hydroxycitrate to two genetically obese hyperlipidemic rodent strains (the Zucker rat and the C57BL/6J-ob/ob mouse) reduced significantly the elevated serum triglyceride levels. The effects of (-)-hydroxycitrate on serum cholesterol levels have not yet been examined in detail.

B. BODY FAT STORES

It was important to ascertain how the chronic administration of (-)-hydroxycitrate would affect the rat's metabolic pattern of lipid accumulation and storage. Studies

---

Fig. 6 continued. before sacrifice as described in the legend of Fig. 4. Data are expressed as nmoles (^{14}C) alanine, nmoles (^{14}C) acetate, μmoles $^{3}H_2O$ or μmoles (^{3}H) acetate converted into fatty acids per g liver per 30 minutes. The vertical bar gives the SE of the mean.
$*p < 0.05$. $**p < 0.01$.

CHOLESTEROL SYNTHESIS IN THE FASTED RAT

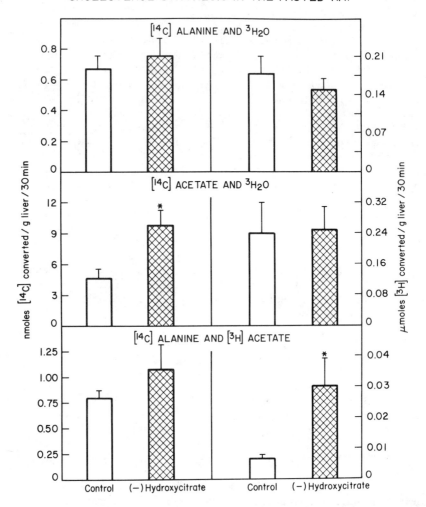

Fig. 7. Influence of (-)-hydroxycitrate on cholesterol synthesis from several precursors in the fasted rat. Six groups of 6 to 9 rats each were prefasted 48 hours, then meal-fed the G-70 diet for 6 to 9 days. They were then administered saline or (-)-hydroxycitrate by stomach tube 21 hours after the last meal. Livers were assayed for in vivo rates of cholesterol synthesis 3 hours later. Radiolabeled precursors were given intravenously 30 minutes before sacrifice as described in the legend of Fig. 4. Data are expressed as nmoles (^{14}C) alanine, nmoles (^{14}C) acetate
Fig. 7 legend continued on next page.

were designed to examine weight gain, appetite, and total body lipid profiles in conjunction with *in vivo* rates of lipid synthesis (Sullivan *et al.*, 1974b). As demonstrated in Table V, the chronic oral administration of certain doses of (-)-hydroxycitrate for 11 days to growing rats produced a significant depression in weight gain and food consumption compared to saline-treated controls. These reductions were reflected metabolically in significant decreases in total body lipid. It was apparent from these data that b.i.d. administration increased significantly the effectiveness of (-)-hydroxycitrate. Subsequent studies on the effect of *ad libitum* feeding, a diet containing (-)-hydroxycitrate, to mature fat rats (6 to 14 months of age) demonstrated similar reductions in appetite, weight gain, and body lipid.

Pair-feeding studies proved that these effects upon weight and body lipids were due to the decreased caloric intake which resulted from (-)-hydroxycitrate treatment. Figure 12 demonstrates that when the food intake of rats in the saline-treated group (paired control) was restricted to the exact quantity consumed by their (-)-hydroxycitrate-treated pair, an equivalent reduction in weight gain was observed. There were no significant differences between the weight gained or food consumed in the (-)-hydroxy-citrate-treated and paired control groups, but both were significantly less than controls at each time interval. Table VI indicates that the body lipid levels of these rats were significantly less than controls in the (-)-hydroxy-citrate-treated and the pair-fed controls. These data demonstrated that the effect of (-)-hydroxycitrate on body lipid levels was due to caloric restriction. Liver lipid levels were identical in the control and treated groups. *In vivo* rates of lipid synthesis were decreased significantly only in the (-)-hydroxycitrate-treated group.

To exclude the possibility that the anorectic effect of (-)-hydroxycitrate was due to a nonspecific tricarboxylate effect, a comparison was made between the effects of the chronic oral administration of citrate (Na_3) and

Fig. 7 continued. μmoles ^3H_2O or μmoles (^3H) acetate converted into cholesterol per g liver per 30 minutes. The vertical bar gives the SE of the mean. *$p < 0.05$. **$p < 0.01$.

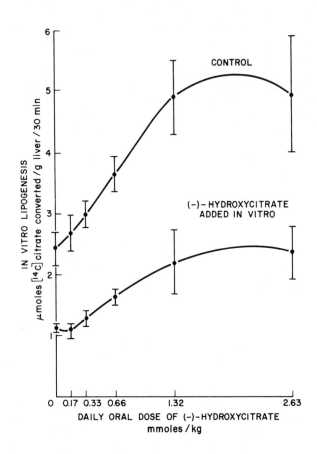

Fig. 8. In vitro rate of hepatic lipogenesis in rats administered (-)-hydroxycitrate orally for 30 days. Rats were prefasted 48 hours, then meal-fed the G-70 diet for 5 days. From day 6 to 36, they received saline or varying concentrations of (-)-hydroxycitrate 1 hour before feeding. On day 36, livers from 4 rats in each group were assayed for in vitro rates of lipogenesis in 10 mM citrate. The upper curve demonstrates the observed rate of lipogenesis; the lower curve gives the rate of lipogenesis when 1 mM (-)-hydroxycitrate was added to each assay. The vertical bar gives the SE of the mean. From Sullivan et al. (1974a). Reprinted by courtesy of the American Oil Chemists' Society.

(-)-hydroxycitrate (Na$_3$). Tabel VII demonstrates that rats treated for 11 days with citrate (Na$_3$) gained significantly more weight than saline controls. Their cumulative

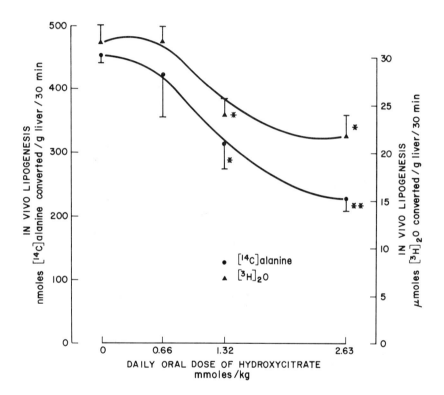

Fig. 9. Reduction of the in vivo rate of hepatic lipogenesis in rats administered (-)-hydroxycitrate orally for 30 days. Rats were prefasted 48 hours, then meal-fed the G-70 diet for 5 days. From day 6 to 36, they received saline or varying concentrations of (-)-hydroxycitrate 1 hour before feeding. On day 36, 8 to 10 rat livers per group were assayed for in vivo lipogenic rates 3 hours after the initiation of feeding. The vertical bar gives the SE of the mean. *p < 0.05. **p < 0.01. From Sullivan et al. (1974a). Reprinted by courtesy of the American Oil Chemists' Society.

food intake and body lipid levels were not significantly different. However, when an equimolar concentration of

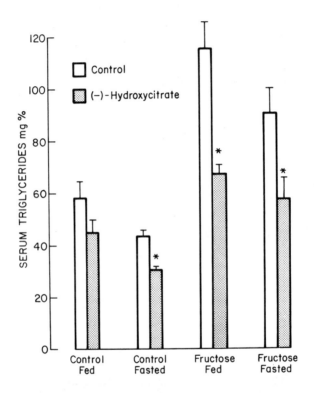

*Fig. 10. Effect of (-)-hydroxycitrate on serum triglycer-ide levels in fed or fasted normotriglyceridemic or hyper-triglyceridemic (fructose-induced) rats. Four groups of 7 rats each were prefasted 48 hours, then meal-fed the G-70 diet for 8 days. On day 9, they were given 10% fruc-tose in the drinking water or plain water immediately be-fore the meal and on day 10 they were either fed or fasted. Rats were administered saline or (-)-hydroxycitrate (1.32 mmoles/kg) by stomach tube at 3 intervals during the period of ± fructose availability which extended over 28 hours: 1) immediately before the meal on day 9 defined as hour 0, 2) at hour 9, and 3) at hour 24. Triglyceride levels (mg %) were determined in serum at hour 28. The vertical bar gives the SE of the mean. *p < 0.05.*

(-)-hydroxycitrate (Na$_3$) was given, a significant reduction
in weight gain and body lipid was observed. Food consumption also was decreased. No differences in liver weight or
liver lipid were detected in either treatment group. *In
vivo* rates of lipid synthesis were unchanged in the citrate
(Na$_3$) group, but significantly inhibited in the rats receiving (-)-hydroxycitrate (Na$_3$).

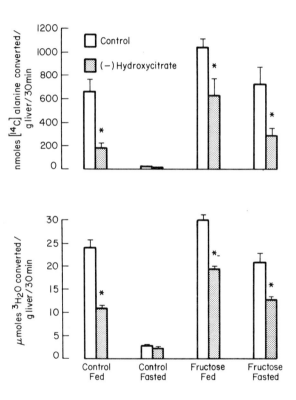

Fig. 11. Effect of (-)-hydroxycitrate on the in vivo *rate
of hepatic fatty acid synthesis in fed or fasted normotriglyceridemic or hypertriglyceridemic (fructose-induced)
rats. See legend of Fig. 10 for details. Livers were assayed for* in vivo *rates of fatty acid synthesis at hour 28.
Data are expressed as nmoles (^{14}C) alanine and μmoles ^3H_2O
converted into fatty acids per g liver per 30 minutes. The
vertical bar gives the SE of the mean.
p < 0.05.

Experiments are currently in progress to ascertain whether the (-)-hydroxycitrate mediated anorexia is related directly, indirectly or not at all to the alteration in metabolic flux produced by this compound. One approach that is being followed is based on the hypothesis that if (-)-hydroxycitrate can penetrate the blood-brain barrier, then an inhibition of brain ATP citrate lyase could result.

Table V

Effect of Oral Administration of (-)-Hydroxycitrate for 11 Days
on Total Weight Gain, Food Consumption and Body Lipid [a] [b]

Daily oral dose of (-)-hydroxycitrate mmoles/kg	Weight gain		Food consumption		Body lipid [c]		
	g [d]	% of control	g [d]	% of control	g [d]	% of carcass weight [d]	% of control [d]
0	12 ± 3		102 ± 3		9.97 ± 0.96	5.7 ± 0.5	
0.66	12 ± 3	100	94 ± 6	92	9.46 ± 0.71	5.5 ± 0.4	96
0.33 b.i.d.	6 ± 2	50	89 ± 3 *	87	6.77 ± 0.82 *	4.1 ± 0.5 *	70
2.63	1 ± 2 **	8	89 ± 3 *	87	6.01 ± 0.31 **	3.5 ± 0.1 **	61
1.32 b.i.d.	2 ± 3 *	17	85 ± 4 *	83	6.34 ± 0.64 **	4.0 ± 0.4 *	67

[a] Reproduced from Sullivan et al. (1974b) by kind permission of the Cambridge University Press.

[b] Five groups of 9 rats each were prefasted 48 hr, then meal-fed the G-70 diet for 5 days. They were then given saline or (—)-hydroxycitrate by stomach tube 1 hr before feeding (and 4 hr after the completion of the meal where b.i.d. administration is indicated) for 11 days.

[c] Body lipid minus liver and blood lipid was determined.

[d] Each value is the group mean ± SE.

* $p < 0.05$ ** $p < 0.01$

This would produce a decreased acetyl CoA pool, thus affecting acetylcholine production. An alteration in acetylcholine levels or rates of turnover could affect cholinergic receptor systems that may be involved in feeding behaviour. Another approach that is being examined is the effect of (-)-hydroxycitrate in systems where either the appetite or the lipogenic status of the animal has been altered.

Summary

(-)-Hydroxycitrate interfered with the conversion of carbohydrate and its metabolites into lipid by inhibiting

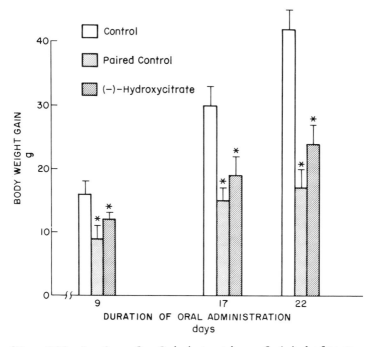

Fig. 12. Effect of oral administration of (-)-hydroxy-citrate for 22 days in a pair-feeding study. Rats were prefasted 48 hours, then meal-fed the G-70 diet for 7 days. They were then divided into 3 groups of 10 and were administered saline (control and paired control) or (-)-hydroxy-citrate (1.32 mmoles/kg) directly before feeding and 4 hours after the completion of the meal. The paired-control group was pair-fed to the (-)-hydroxycitrate-treated rats. The vertical bar gives the SE of the mean. *P < 0.05. From Sullivan et al. (1974b). Reprinted courtesy of the American Oil Chemists' Society.

significantly *in vivo* rates of fatty acid and cholesterol synthesis through its activity as a potent competitive inhibitor of ATP citrate lyase, the enzyme generating acetyl CoA in the cytoplasm. These effects of (-)-hydroxycitrate on *in vivo* lipid biosynthesis were similar after acute and chronic administration. The other isomers of hydroxy-citrate were ineffective in significantly altering lipid synthesis. (-)-Hydroxycitrate activated acetyl CoA carbox-ylase *in vivo* only in the fasted state.

Table VI

Body Lipid Levels of Rats Pair-fed to
(-)-Hydroxycitrate—treated Rats for 22 Days [a]

| Treatment [b] | Body lipid [c] | | Liver lipid |
	% of carcass weight	% of control	% of liver weight
Control	5.1 ± 0.5		3.2 ± 0.0
Pair-fed control	3.4 ± 0.4 *	67	3.1 ± 0.0
(-)-Hydroxycitrate	3.8 ± 0.3 *	75	3.1 ± 0.0

[a] Reproduced from Sullivan et al. (1974b) by kind permission of the Cambridge University Press.

[b] Three groups of 10 rats were prefasted 48 hr, then meal-fed the G-70 diet for 5 days. The control groups were then administered saline and the experimental group received (—)-hydroxycitrate (1.32 mmoles/kg b.i.d.) directly before feeding and 4 hr after the completion of the meal for 22 days. During this time the pair-fed controls received the exact quantity of food that the (—)-hydroxycitrate-treated rats had consumed on the previous day.

[c] Body lipid minus blood and liver lipid was determined.

[d] Each value is the group mean ± SE.

* $p < 0.05$

The extent of the diversion of carbohydrate carbons from lipid synthesis by (-)-hydroxycitrate was considerable since it persisted in the liver for the entire period during which control animals exhibited significant lipogenic rates and occurred in the 3 major lipogenic tissues (adipose, liver, and small intestine). Some of the carbons diverted from hepatic lipid biosynthesis were channeled into glycogen. Respiration, phosphorylation, ketone body formation, and urinary glucose excretion were unchanged by (-)-hydroxycitrate administration.

(-)-Hydroxycitrate reduced significantly the accumulation of lipid in body fat stores and in blood. Body lipid levels were depressed due to a significant reduction in appetite, as proved by pair-feeding studies. These effects on appetite, weight gain, and body lipid levels were demonstrated in growing lean and mature fat rats. However, the administration of citrate under the same experimental

Table VII

Comparison of the Effect of Oral Administration of Citrate (Na)$_3$ and
(-)-Hydroxycitrate (Na)$_3$ for 11 Days [a]

Treatment [b]	Weight gain g [d]	Weight gain % of control	Food consumption g [d]	Body lipid [b] g [d]	Body lipid [b] % of carcass weight [d]	Body lipid [b] % of control	Liver weight g [d]	Liver lipid % of liver weight [d]
Saline	20 ± 3		120 ± 5	7.4 ± 1.0	4.5 ± 0.7		5.8 ± 0.3	3.2 ± 0.1
Citrate (Na)$_3$	27 ± 2 *	135	131 ± 5	6.8 ± 0.8	4.1 ± 0.5	92	5.9 ± 0.2	3.2 ± 0.1
(-)-Hydroxy-citrate (Na)$_3$	12 ± 2 *	60	112 ± 4	4.4 ± 0.5 *	2.9 ± 0.5 *	62	5.8 ± 0.2	2.9 ± 0.1

[a] Reproduced from Sullivan et al. (1974b) by kind permission of the Cambridge University Press.

[b] Three groups of 14 rats each were prefasted 48 hr, then meal-fed the G-70 diet for 5 days. They were then administered saline, citrate (Na)$_3$ (1.32 mmoles/kg) or (—)-hydroxycitrate (Na)$_3$ (1.32 mmoles/kg) 1 hr before feeding and 4 hr after completion of the meal for 11 days.

[c] Body lipid minus liver and blood lipid was determined.

[d] Each value is the group mean ± SE.

* $p < 0.05$

conditions had no effect on food intake, weight gain, body lipid levels or hepatic lipid biosynthesis. Serum triglycerides were significantly reduced when (-)-hydroxycitrate was given to the hypertriglyceridemic-fructose rat.

ACKNOWLEDGMENTS

The studies reported here were conducted with the excellent collaboration of my scientific colleagues, J. Triscari, J. G. Hamilton, O. N. Miller, and R. W. Guthrie. The expert technical assistance of G. Mackie and the synthesis of the hydroxycitrates by R. W. Guthrie and R. W. Kierstead were invaluable.

References

Barth, C., Sladek, M., and Decker, K. (1971). *Biochim. Biophys. Acta* 248, 24.
Barth, C., Hackenschmidt, J., Ullmann, H., and Decker, K. (1972a). *FEBS Letters* 22, 343.

Barth, C., Sladek, M., and Decker, K. (1972b). *Biochim. Biophys. Acta* 260, 1.

Bhaduri, A., and Srere, P. A. (1963). *Biochim. Biophys. Acta* 70, 221.

Boll, P. M., Sørensen, E., and Balieu, E. (1969). *Acta Chem. Scan.* 23, 286.

Brunengraber, H., and Lowenstein, J. M. (1973). *FEBS Letters* 36, 130.

Brunengraber, H., Sabine, J. R., Boutry, M., and Lowenstein, J. M. (1972). *Arch. Biochem. Biophys.* 150, 392.

Cahn, R. S., Ingold, C. K., and Prelog, V. (1956). *Experimentia* 12, 81.

Cheema-Dhadli, S., Halperin, M. L., and Leznoff, C. C. (1973). *Eur. J. Biochem.* 38, 98.

Cram, D. J., and Elhafes, F. A. A. (1952). *J. Amer. Chem. Soc.* 74, 5828.

D'Adamo, A. F., Jr., and Haft, D. E. (1965). *J. Biol. Chem.* 240, 613.

Daikuhara, Y., Tsunemi, T., and Takeda, Y. (1968). *Biochim. Biophys. Acta* 158, 51.

Decker, K., and Barth, C. (1973). *Mol. and Cell. Biochem.* 2, 179.

Fritz, I. B., and Yue, K. T. N. (1964). *Am. J. Physiol.* 206, 531.

Glusker, J. P. (1971). *The Enzymes* 5, 413.

Glusker, J. P., and Srere, P. A. (1973). *Biorganic Chem.* 2, 301.

Glusker, J. P., Minkin, J. A., Casciato, C. A., and Soule, F. B. (1969). *Arch. Biochem. Biophys.* 13, 573.

Goodridge, A. (1973). *J. Biol. Chem.* 248, 4318.

Gregolin, C., Ryder, E., Kleinschmidt, A. K., Warner, R. C., and Lane, M. D. (1966a). *Proc. Natl. Acad. Sci.* 56, 148.

Gregolin, C., Ryder, E., Warner, R. C., Kleinschmidt, A. K., and Lane, M. D. (1966b). *Proc. Natl. Acad. Sci.* 56, 1751.

Gregolin, C., Ryder, E., Warner, R. C., Kleinschmidt, A. K., Chang, H., and Lane, M. D. (1968). *J. Biol. Chem.* 243, 4236.

Griebel, C. (1939). *Chem. Abst.* 33, 7491.

Griebel, C. (1942). *Chem. Abst.* 37, 4704.

Hackenschmidt, J., Barth, C., and Decker, K. (1972). *FEBS Letters* 27, 131.

Hashimoto, T., and Numa, S. (1971). *Eur. J. Biochem.* 18, 319.

Horikawa, K., and Masuyama, S. (1965). *Yukagaku* 14, 179.

Inoue, H., Suzuki, F., Fukunishi, K., Adachi, K., and
    Takeda, Y. (1966). *J. Biochem. Tokyo* 60, 543.
Jungas, R. L. (1968). *Biochemistry* 7, 3708.
Kornacker, M. S., and Lowenstein, J. M. (1965). *Biochem.
    J.* 94, 209.
Lane, M. D., Moss, J., Ryder, E., and Stoll, E. (1971).
    Advan. Enzyme Regul. 9, 237.
Lardy, H. A. (1966). *Harvey Lectures* 60, 261.
Lewis, Y. S. (1969). *In* "Methods in Enzymology" (J. M.
    Lowenstein, ed.), p. 613. Academic Press, New York.
Lewis, Y. S., and Neelakantan, S. (1965). *Phytochem.* 4,
    619.
Lewis, Y. S., Neelakantan, S., and Anjanamurthy, C.
    (1964). *Curr. Sci.* 3, 82.
von Lippmann, E. (1883). *Ber. Chem. Ges.* 16, 1078.
Lowenstein, J. M. (1968). *In* "Metabolic Roles of Citrate"
    (T. W. Goodwin, ed.), p. 61. Academic Press, New York.
Lowenstein, J. M. (1970). *In* "Essays in Cell Metabolism"
    (W. Bartley, H. L. Kornberg, and J. R. Quayle, eds.),
    p. 153. John Wiley and Sons, Ltd., London.
Lowenstein, J. M. (1971). *J. Biol. Chem.* 246, 629.
Martin, D. B., and Vagelos, P. R. (1962). *J. Biol. Chem.*
    237, 1787.
Martins, C., and Maue, R. (1941). *Physiol. Chemie* 269, 33.
Matsuhashi, M., Matsuhashi, S., and Lynen, F. (1964).
    Biochem. Z. 340, 263.
Rous, S. (1971). *FEBS Letters* 12, 338.
Rous, S. (1974). *Biochimie* 56, 153.
Rous, S., and Favarger, P. (1973). *FEBS Letters* 37, 231.
Spencer, A. F., and Lowenstein, J. M. (1962). *J. Biol.
    Chem.* 237, 3640.
Srere, P. A. (1972). *In* "Current Topics in Cellular
    Regulation" (B. L. Horecker, and E. R. Stadtman, eds.),
    p. 229. Academic Press, New York.
Srere, P. A., and Bhaduri, A. (1962). *Biochim. Biophys.
    Acta* 59, 487.
Start, C., and Newsholme, E. A. (1968). *Biochem. J.* 107,
    411.
Sullivan, A. C. (1973). Ph.D. Thesis University Micro-
    films, Ann Arbor, Michigan.
Sullivan, A. C., Miller, O. N., Wittman, J. S., and
    Hamilton, J. G. (1971). *J. Nutrition* 101, 265.
Sullivan, A. C., Hamilton, J. G., Miller, O. N., and
    Wheatley, V. R. (1972). *Arch. Biochem. Biophys.* 150,
    183.
Sullivan, A. C., Triscari, J., Hamilton, J. G., Miller, O.
    N., and Wheatley, V. R. (1974a). *Lipids* 9, 121.

Sullivan, A. C., Triscari, J., Hamilton, J. G., and Miller, O. N. (1974b). *Lipids* 9, 129.

Sullivan, A. C., Triscari, J., and Miller, O. N. (1974c). *Federation Proceedings* 33, 650.

Sullivan, A. C., Triscari, J., Hamilton, J. G., Miller, O. N., and Ontko, J. A. (1974d). *The Pharmacologist* 16, 315.

Vagelos, P. R., Alberts, A. W., and Martin, D. B. (1963). *J. Biol. Chem.* 238, 533.

Waite, M., and Wakil, S. J. (1962). *J. Biol. Chem.* 237, 2750.

Watson, J. A., and Lowenstein, J. M. (1970). *J. Biol. Chem.* 245, 5993.

Watson, J. A., Fang, M., and Lowenstein, J. M. (1969). *Arch. Biochem. Biophys.* 135, 209.

Wheatley, V. R., Kumarisiri, M., and Brind, J. L. (1973). *J. Invest. Derm.* 61, 357.

Early Nutritional Influences on
Development

M. R. C. GREENWOOD

I.   Introduction

The quality of life, measured by the availability of
the appropriate quantity and quality of nutrients during
early development, may have profound consequences for the
mature adult. Internationally, the distribution of nutrients, like the distribution of wealth, is disproportionate.
Some countries like the United States and Western Europe have
a superabundance of crops and technology while most of the
African and South American countries have vast undernour-
ished populations. This inequality in the availability of
nutrients has confronted scientists interested in early development, physiology, and nutrition with two seemingly different pathologies resulting from early infant nutrition:
malnutrition on the one hand, and obesity on the other.
While seemingly quite opposite sides of the early nutritional experience, they share the common ground that in both
cases the normal orderly sequence of cellular proliferation
and differentiation is disrupted. Restriction of the early
diet either by total calorie deprivation or by deficiencies
in vitamins, minerals, or protein results in a mature organism that has been permanently stunted. If malnutrition
is imposed early and maintained throughout the suckling
period in rats, and for approximately 18-24 months in man,
"catch-up" growth is incomplete. Although many organs and
tissues are especially affected by early dietary deficiencies, two of those carefully studied have been adipose tissue, that tissue in which size is most readily influenced by
fluctuation in caloric consumption and the brain, in which
size is perhaps the least affected, but in which function
is of paramount concern.

Interest in the permanent effects of infant malnutrition is worldwide, and of particular concern are the effects

of malnutrition on brain function. Since the original work by Winick and Noble (1966) demonstrating that brain cell number was affected by early malnutrition in rats, concern over the importance of early rehabilitation and the "critical" timing of such efforts has mounted. Several laboratories studying malnutrition are attempting to establish the extent of brain cellular damage during gestation and early lactation and to determine how long and how soon rehabilitation is effective.

In recent years, a very different problem has come to the forefront in respect to health-related societal cares: the fact that in a nation such as the United States, where food is generally abundant and readily attainable, some 30% of the adult population can be classified as obese, i.e., more than 20% above ideal body weight. Questions regarding the obese condition have begun to focus upon the effects of early infant overnutrition and the potential for adult hypercellular obesity, because of the well-known clinical observations that children who are visibly obese by age two are likely to be obese as adults. Furthermore, clinicians have observed for years that individuals who have been obese since childhood have a high rate of recidivism. Although it had been reported (Hellman *et al.*, 1962) that adipose cell number was increased in genetically obese mice, it was not until the method of Coulter counting of osmium fixed fat cells was developed by Hirsch and Gallian (1968) that extensive studies on the cellular state of obese humans was undertaken.

Using this technique, Jules Hirsch and his colleagues showed that very obese individuals had a remarkably elevated fat cell number and that all obese individuals had increased fat cell sizes (Hirsch and Knittle, 1970). Furthermore, their data strongly suggested that the earlier the age of onset of the obesity, the more likely the obese individual was to be hypercellular (Hirsch and Knittle, 1970). Such findings have served to focus interest on the events surrounding an organism's early nutritional status.

II. Human Studies: Adipose Cellularity and Weight Reduction

Although only minimal data are available on the normal development of adipose cellularity in humans, the few existing studies suggest that once the adult fat cell number is attained, new cells are not formed, and fat cell turnover is minimal, if it occurs at all. The evidence for this position is that (a) after weight reduction obese, adult, hypercellular individuals maintain the same adipocyte number and show only a reduced cell size (Hirsch and Knittle, 1970; Stern *et al.*, 1972); (b) when normal volunteers were asked to increase body weight, no increases in fat cell number were noted, but cells became enlarged, and upon weight reduction only cell size changed (Sims *et al.*, 1968); and (c) the little developmental data that exist suggest that normal humans form fat cells postnatally up to two years of age and perhaps again at puberty (Knittle, personal communication).

III. Animal Studies: Normal Development

Before it was possible to assess the effect of early nutritional influences on adult adipose tissue cellularity in animal models, it was necessary to determine the normal course of cellular development in this tissue. In the normal Sprague-Dawley rat, the number of adipocytes in the epididymal fat pad increases from birth to 12-14 weeks of age (Fig. 1). The pattern of development that is seen in the epididymal fat pad has been shown by Johnson *et al.* (1971) to also be characteristic of other fat depots in lean rats and mice, e.g., retroperitoneal, subcutaneous, and perimetrial (Fig. 2).

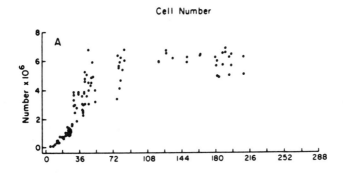

Fig. 1. Legend on next page.

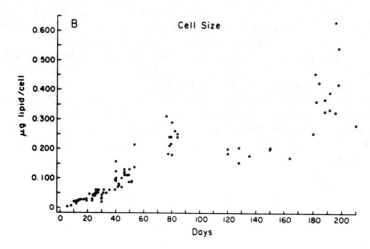

Fig. 1. Cellularity of rat epididymal fat pad. For both cell number and size, each data point represents the mean or pooled data value for 4-12 rats. From J. Lipid Res. 15, 476 (1974).

Once the adult cell number has been attained, dietary manipulation or production of gross obesity by electrolytic lesions of the ventromedial hypothalamus (VMH) in the postpubertal rat affect only the fat cell size and do not change fat cell number. However, when nutritional status is manipulated before the end of the suckling period, it is possible to change the ultimate number of adult fat cells. To produce an alteration in cellularity through postnatal nutritional status, the classic design of McCance and Widdowson (1962) was utilized by Knittle and Hirsch (1968). Knittle and Hirsch manipulated nutritional status from birth by forming litters of 22 pups per mother ("large litters") and litters of 4 pups per mother ("small litters"). Such a manipulation produced heavier than normal pups from the "small litters" and lighter than normal pups from the "large litters." The early nutritional deprivation experienced by the pups in large litters affected the normal growth and development of numerous organs including the brain. The effect on adipose tissue cellularity is a permanent reduction in adipocyte number which cannot be reversed by nutritional rehabilitation after weaning. The effect of early overnutrition on fat cell number was convincingly shown by Lemmonier (1972) in a series of experiments in which mice were fed a high fat diet during gestation and lactation. When the high fat diet was fed in this fashion, the offspring

DEVELOPMENT OF
ADIPOSE CELL NUMBER

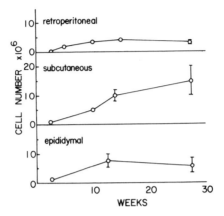

Fig. 2. Cellularity of retroperitoneal, subcutaneous, and epididymal fat depots in nonobese Zucker rats. Redrawn from data of Johnson, J. Lipid Res. 12, 706 (1971).

were obese and had a significantly increased fat cell number as adults.

These findings in rodents led to a peculiar paradox which has been discussed in relation to the human studies as well (Widdowson and Shaw, 1973). When Coulter counting of osmium fixed cells or visual estimation of fat cells is employed, fat cell counts increase after birth until approximately 12-14 weeks, the time of puberty in the rat (Hirsch and Han, 1969; Greenwood and Hirsch, 1974) (see Fig. 1). Although fat cells appear continuously from weaning until puberty when such counting techniques are employed, the early nutritional manipulation experiments demonstrated that dietary restriction after weaning and before puberty does not permanently change the organism's ability to attain the normal adult fat cell number when *ad libitum* feeding is reinstated (Hirsch and Han, 1969).

The explanation advanced for this apparent paradox suggested that all the fat cells seen in the adult rat epididymal pad were formed before or during the suckling period, but that some continued to fill with lipid and reach countable size between weaning until the onset of puberty. Until recently, this explanation had not been substantiated experimentally. The hypothesis that fat cells are synthesized at

some point early in development, but differentiate and fill
with lipid for a much longer period and possibly throughout
life, presupposed the existence of "preadipocytes." Such
"preadipocytes" would appear morphologically like fibroblasts containing little, if any, lipid, but would be pro-
gramed with the potential for synthesis of the cellular
machinery needed for rapid lipid accumulation. Unfortunately, the existent techniques for counting fat cells depend upon the cells containing a certain critical amount of
lipid, and, therefore, the existence of "preadipocytes" cannot be assessed with these methods.

IV. Animal Studies: ^{3}H-Thymidine *In Vivo* Injections

Resolution of this seeming paradox has recently been
accomplished with a series of ^{3}H-thymidine incorporation
experiments in normal rats. Rats ranging from nine days to
five months of age were injected intraperitoneally with ^{3}H-
thymidine. The ^{3}H-thymidine was incorporated into all cells
undergoing DNA synthesis at the time of the injection. Included in this category of proliferating cells would be any
nonlipid-laden "preadipocytes." Therefore, in developing
adipose tissue all "preadipocytes" engaged in DNA synthesis
would become radioactively labeled. As they differentiated
and filled with lipid at some later point in development,
the label would serve to identify them as the precursor cells
synthesized at the time of the thymidine injection. Using a
modification of the collagenase digestion, fat cell isolation procedure developed by Rodbell (1964) and described
elsewhere (Greenwood and Hirsch, 1974), we were able to
prepare two cell fractions from adipose tissue: a stromal-
vascular fraction and an adipocyte fraction. The stromal-
vascular fraction consisted of cells from the vascular bed,
macrophages, leucocytes, and, of course, "preadipocytes."
The adipocyte fraction consisted of isolated differentiated
fat cells. Both fractions appeared free of contamination
with either lipid or stroma, respectively, at the light
microscopic level. By utilizing this fractionation technique, the two cell pools from rats of various ages were
prepared at specified intervals. Since it is well known
(Napolitano, 1965) that mature fat cells are not mitotic,
one would predict that all the radioactivity would be contained in the stromal-vascular fraction and not in the
isolated fat cell fraction, when the rats were killed and
their tissue cells separated shortly after isotope injection. With the passage of time after injection, the nonlipid-laden preadipocytes could be expected to fill with

lipid. As animals were killed and cells harvested at various time intervals after injection, one would predict that radioactivity-labeled cells would begin to appear in the isolated fat cell fraction. Utilization of these methods enables one to observe changes in the specific activity (dpms/µgDNA) of both cell fractions which reflect the differentiation of "preadipocytes" into mature adipocytes, after the labeling of preadipocytes during proliferation. DNA was determined using a modification of the Kissane and Robbins fluorometric technique and is described elsewhere (Greenwood and Hirsch, 1974).

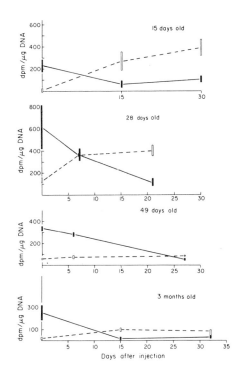

Fig. 3. In vivo injection of (3-H) thymidine; specific activity of adipocyte and stromal fractions. Open bars and dotted lines represent the specific activity determined at various times post injection in the isolated adipocyte fraction. Closed bars and solid lines represent the specific activity determined in the stromal-vascular fraction. Bars represent the ranges of the two pools sampled at each time point. From J. Lipid Res. *15, 478 (1974).*

The results obtained when ^{3}H-thymidine was injected
into rats 15 days, 28 days, 49 days, and 3 months of age
are shown in Fig. 3. In all cases, it should be noted that
the specific activity of the stromal-vascular cell pool
declined over time, after injection of the isotope. In rats
injected with isotope at 15 and 28 days of age, the specific
activity of the fat cell fraction increased over time, indicating that precursor fat cells labeled on day 15 or 28
were filling with lipid and being counted in the mature fat
cell fraction. In rats injected at 49 days of age, a slight
increase in the specific activity of the mature fat cell
fraction was seen, but the pattern was less pronounced than
at 15 and 28 days of age. In the rats injected at 3 months
of age, a similar pattern in specific activity was noted.
Another study of 22 day, 35 day, and 5 month old rats re-
vealed that 22 day old rats displayed a pattern similar to
15 and 28 day old rats; 35 day old rats showed a pattern
similar to 49 day old rats, and 5 month old rats appeared
to be similar to 3 month old rats (Greenwood and Hirsch,
1974). These results may be more clearly illustrated from
a study of the accumulation of radioactivity in the fat cell
fraction (Fig. 4). In rats injected with isotope at 15 and
28 days of age, two processes are apparent: (a) fat cells
are synthesized on day 15 or 28 and (b) most of the cells
synthesized remain undifferentiated and can take considerable lengths of time (30 days or more) to differentiate and
fill with enough lipid to be isolated as mature fat cells.
In rats injected with isotope at 49 days of age, some new
fat cells were made as reflected by the increase of label in
adipocyte DNA. However, the newly made precursor cells do
not remain undifferentiated for long, but rather appear as
mature cells after 2-6 days, confirming the earlier report
of Hollenberg and Vost (1968). Since there is no net change
in adipocyte DNA radioactive label in 3 month old rats, one
can conclude that no "precursor" cells are being made and
filled with lipid. These isotope incorporation studies
have led to the conclusion that there are three periods of
postnatal growth in rat epididymal fat (Fig. 5). There is
a period after birth until weaning characterized primarily
by proliferation with differentiation and lipid filling as a
less prominent feature. From weaning until approximately
sexual maturity in the rat, some small amount of fat cell
proliferation may occur, but tissue growth is predominantly
a result of lipid filling of existent cells. The final period of tissue growth is accomplished by adipose cellular
enlargement only (see Fig. 2).

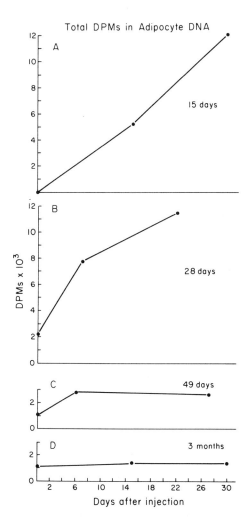

Fig. 4. Total dpms in adipocyte DNA for 15 day old, 28 day
old, 49 day old, and 3 month old rats. Each data point
represents the mean value for the two pools sampled at each
time. From J. Lipid Res. 15, 479 (1974).

Cell Number Development

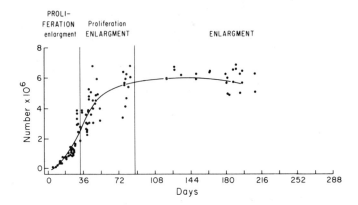

Fig. 5. *Development of fat cellularity in epididymal fat. Periods indicated by vertical lines represent the course of fat cell proliferation as determined by ^3H-thymidine incorporation into fat cell DNA.*

V. Animal Studies: Genetically Obese Zucker Rats

In contrast to the normal Sprague-Dawley rat, when fat cells are counted in the Zucker obese rat (fa/fa), the numbers continue to increase well beyond 12-14 weeks of age. This increase in number, although observed in all adipose depots, is best demonstrated in the subcutaneous depot fat (Johnson *et al.*, 1973) (see Fig. 6). The pattern of proliferation of adipocytes as elucidated by ^3H-thymidine injection has not yet been reported, although the studies are currently in progress. In order to determine if Zucker obese rats, like Sprague-Dawley rats, respond to early nutritional manipulation by showing changes in adult fat cell number, Zucker rats were raised from birth in large (19 pups), small (4 pups), and standard (8 pups) litters. It was apparent that during the suckling period, expression of the obese gene was masked by the nutritional manipulation. Body weights of the rats reflected the nutritional treatment: rats raised in "small" litters were heavier than rats raised in standard litters and conversely, rats raised in "large" litters were lighter than rats raised in control litters (Fig. 7). However, when the rats were allowed to feed

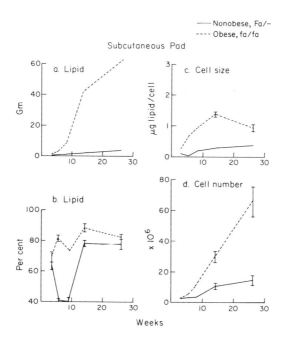

Fig. 6. Grams of lipid (a), percentage of lipid (b), cell size (c), and cell number (d) of the subcutaneous fat depot in Zucker obese (fa/fa) and nonobese (Fa/e) rats. For all groups n=6. Critical data points are plotted as mean values ± SEM. In some cases, the SEM was too small to be accurately indicated on the scale used. From J. Lipid Res. 12, 706 (1971).

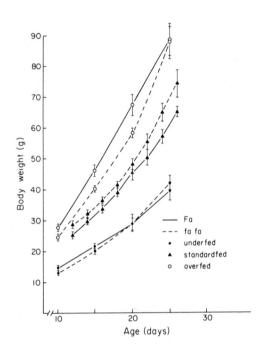

Fig. 7. *Preweaning growth of Zucker obese and nonobese
rats. Effect of over-, under-, and* ad libitum *feeding.
Values are mean ± SEM.* From J. of Nutr. *103, 740 (1973).*

ad libitum from weaning until the termination of the experiment at 26 weeks of age a very different pattern emerged.
All genetically obese rats (fa/fa) were significantly
heavier than all lean rats (Fa/-), regardless of the early
nutritional manipulation. The effect of the litter-size
manipulation is, however, apparent. Within the obese rat
population, those raised in "small" litters were heavier
than those raised in standard litters and those raised in
"large" litters were lighter. A similar effect was seen
among the lean rats (Fig. 8). When total adipose tissue
cellularity was determined, however, a surprising and in-
triguing finding emerged. As predicted by the difference in
body weights, all obese (fa/fa) rats have more fat cells

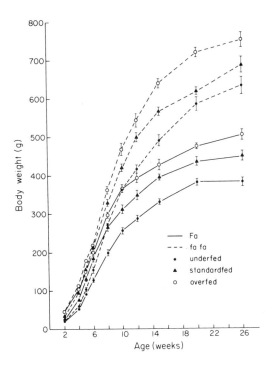

Fig. 8. Postweaning growth of Zucker obese and nonobese rats. Effect of under-, over-, and ad libitum *feeding during the preweaning period. Values are mean ± SEM. From J. of* Nutr. *103, 740 (1973).*

than their lean littermates (Fa/-), and the lean rats (Fa/-) displayed a cellularity profile similar to that described by Knittle and Hirsch: underfeeding during infancy decreased fat cell number; overfeeding during infancy increased fat cell number (Fig. 9). The effect of the early litter manipulation on adipose cellularity in the adult

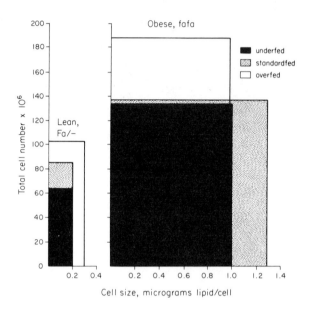

Fig. 9. *Relative contribution of cell size and cell number to total adipose cellularity in the Zucker obese and non-obese rat. From J. Nutr. 103, 741 (1973).*

obese rat (fa/fa) was quite different; however, those obese rats overfed during infancy had a striking increase in fat cell number compared to standard fed obese rats, but under-feeding of the obese rat (fa/fa) failed to reduce adult adipocyte number. Does this mean that the Zucker obese rat has the ability to continue proliferation of adipocytes past the time that proliferation ceases in the lean animal? The presence of the recessive gene *fa* in the homozygous state in this animal model may well regulate growth and the prolif-erative process by extending the normal time course of preadipocyte differentiation and proliferation period, allowing genetically obese rats to "catch-up" or "overgrow" after early nutritional experience. Other hypotheses con-cerning the mechanism by which fat cell number continues to increase post weaning in the Zucker obese rat are also plausible, and a definitive answer must await the outcome of ^{3}H-thymidine incorporation studies in this strain. What does seem clear and may have relevance to the human condition is the observation that in the presence of a genetic predisposition toward obesity, nutritional influences are even more marked, particularly in the direction of still further increases in fat cell hyperplasia. Although the inheritance of obesity in man has never been convincingly shown, several studies have suggested that a correlation exists between parental overweight and incidence of obesity in the offspring (Bauer, 1947; Mayer, 1953). It may be that where the risk for childhood obesity is high, particular attention should be given to using dietary means in maintaining infants and young children at weights considered to be within the normal range for their age and height.

It should be pointed out, at this point, that while this discussion has focused on the number of adipose cells in normal, obese, and nutritionally manipulated rodents and man, the size of the adipocyte is an even more responsive indicator to the nutritional state of the organism. Presumably, in the adult, adipocyte size is controlled as a function of the absolute caloric input and hormonal status. The mechanism of controlling the adipocyte size during normal development is not understood. When obesity occurs after maturity in rats, mice, and humans, tremendous increases in fat cell size are seen without the increase seen in fat cell number during the development of juvenile obesity (Hirsch and Knittle, 1970; Stern *et al.*, 1972, Bjorntorp and Sjostrom, 1971).

VI.   Brain Development: Normal Growth

While in this country, a major problem in pediatric nutrition is the existence of overnutrition and the production of a superabundance of fat cells, presumed to be both esthetically and metabolically undesirable, the problem of undernutrition is much more a part of life in underdeveloped or impoverished parts of the world. Since undernutrition has lasting effects on numerous tissues including adipose tissue, the effects of early nutritional status on the normal acquisition of brain function has aroused much more emotion and concern. Winick has shown that during normal brain development, total DNA content, considered to be an index of total brain cell number, increases in a manner remarkably similar to the pattern seen in adipose tissue, the difference being that brain cellular proliferation takes place predominantly before birth in the human (Fig. 10). Considerable evidence has accumulated to suggest that two peaks of cellular proliferation occur in normal brain. In man,

DNA CONTENT OF NORMAL HUMAN BRAIN

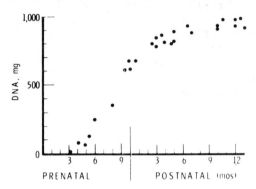

Fig. 10. *Total DNA content of the human brain derived from 27 cases of therapeutic abortions, crib-deaths, accidental deaths, and poisoning. From* Federation Proceedings *29, 1511 (1970).*

these peaks correspond to a prenatal peak around the 26th week of gestational age and a second peak at birth continuing for some time after (Winick, 1970). Similar peak periods of cellular proliferation appear in developing rat brain (Winick and Noble, 1965). In addition, Brasel *et al.* have demonstrated that brain DNA polymerase activity correlates closely with prenatal and postnatal changes in DNA content (Brasel *et al.*, 1970). Both Winick and Brasel have supported the postulate that the DNA polymerase changes reflect the prenatal proliferation of neuronal cells and the postnatal proliferation of glial cells. Of further interest is the established finding that rates of cellular proliferation vary in different parts of the brain (Fish and Winick, 1969). The major effects of nutritional manipulation are most profound in those areas of the brain where cellular proliferation is proceeding most rapidly at the time of the manipulation.

The functional differentiation that occurs during normal brain development includes the laying down of myelin sheaths, which is another form of lipid filling of cells, and which, like adipocyte proliferation and differentiation, proceeds concurrently with neuronal proliferation in an orderly and sequential fashion. Although some of the brain lipid is contained in subcellular organelles, the majority of the lipid is found in the membrane fraction, primarily in myelin sheaths. Therefore, on a gross analysis, changes in total brain lipids could be expected to reflect changes in the degree of neuronal myelination. In humans, 90% of the total lipid is present at 2 years of age with adult values reached by 10 years of age. A fine analysis of the process of myelination requires an analysis of lipid classes. The fatty acid composition of myelin shows marked and varied changes throughout early postnatal development (O'Brien and Sampson, 1965). Cholesterol is present in relatively high concentrations early and slowly rises to still higher concentrations with increasing postnatal age (Rosso et al., 1970). In the rat, the rate of cholesterol deposition is highest postnatally at 15-20 days. This peak corresponds to one week after the postnatal peak of DNA synthesis and signals the onset of myelination. In the adult organism, cholesterol represents the most abundant lipid component of myelin. Cerebrosides which are only marginally detectable at birth begin to appear as myelination commences and their presence has been suggested as essential for the formation of compact myelination (Davison, 1972). In the adult, approximately 90% of the cerebroside present in the brain is contained in the myelin and is required for maintenance of structural integrity (Rathbone, 1965).

VII. Brain Development: Effect of Early Malnutrition

When the nutritional status of rats is manipulated from birth by changing litter size or by further restricting protein by feeding the gestating mother a 6% casein diet, permanent decreases in brain cell DNA occur which are not ameliorated by nutritional rehabilitation; increases in brain cell DNA due to overfeeding have not been reported. When either prenatal (maternal) malnutrition or postnatal (litter manipulation during suckling) is separately imposed, a 15% reduction in total brain cell DNA occurs (Fig. 11). However, when both prenatal and postnatal malnutrition are employed, a striking 40% reduction of brain cell DNA is seen (Fig. 11). This effect of malnutrition has also been demonstrated in human brain DNA by Rosso, Winick, and Brasel (Rathbone, 1965). When the brains of marasmic children of normal birth weight or children with kwashiorkor (both groups representing postnatal malnutrition) were examined after death, they were shown to have a 10-20% reduc-

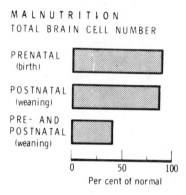

Fig. 11. Comparison of caloric restriction after birth, protein restriction during gestation, and "combined" prenatal and postnatal restriction. From Federation Proceedings *29, 1512 (1970).*

tion in total brain DNA. The brains of children who were both marasmic and of low birth weight (presumably, but not definitively, due to maternal malnutrition) showed a 40% reduction at death in total brain DNA (Fig. 12). The effect

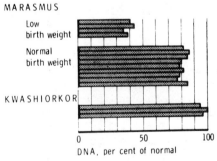

Fig. 12. Total DNA content in brains of children who died of malnutrition. From Federation Proceedings *29, 1513 (1970).*

of the malnutrition was not confined to a reduction in total brain DNA, but was also marked by a reduction in total lipids (Rathbone, 1965). The reduction in total brain lipids was reflected in a depression in total brain cholesterol and phospholipids. Much more complex changes are seen if the fatty acid composition is analyzed (Galli *et al.*, 1970). It seems apparent from these studies, that early caloric deprivation during either cellular proliferation or the early period of myelin formation results in both a decrease in the number of brain cells and their degree of functional differentiation.

One might then ask whether the effects of malnutrition are due to a generalized total caloric restriction or whether more specific dietary deficiencies produce the syndrome or any part of it. Of particular interest is the question of whether diets deficient in essential fatty acids (EFA) produce changes in the central nervous system. One reasons for this particular question is that polyunsaturated essential fatty acids are present in high concentrations as part of the structural constituents of myelin, and diets deficient in EFA early in development might be expected to affect the normal sequential laying down of myelin and to interfere with the acquisition of normal neuronal function. Some insight into this problem may be forthcoming from current work involving total parenteral nutrition. Infants receiving total parenteral nutrition early in life prior to surgical correction of gastrointestinal defects, do not receive any lipid in the infusion. Since it is illegal to administer lipids intravenously in the United States as part of such infusions, individuals on total intravenous alimentation become EFA deficient. The work of White *et al.* (1971) has been of particular interest in this area. In their original study, they showed that when pregnant rats were fed EFA deficient diets and their offspring were continued on the EFA deficient regime, these offspring weighed significantly less and had lighter brains than control rats. Furthermore, there were marked changes in the fatty acid composition of brain lipids, particularly in ethanolamine phosphoglyceride (EPG) fractions. These changes induced by EFA deficiency were initially thought to be reversible by refeeding an EFA containing diet. However, more recent work has indicated that although certain fatty acids attain normal concentration, abnormal concentrations are present even after prolonged rehabilitation.

When the effect of early nutrition has been to reduce brain cell number or degree of myelination, the question of

the functional significance of these effects has been
raised. Several animal experiments have purported to show
that rats receiving total caloric restriction or EFA deficient diets early in life display behavior differences as
adults. While the initial interpretation of these results
led to the suggestion that reduced performance on certain
behavioral tests could be equated with the reduced IQ or
academic performance seen in malnourished children, more
careful analysis of the data has failed to establish this
point. Strong correlations exist, but causality is far
from understood.

Summary

In all biological systems the process of growth and
development after birth is orderly and sequential. Most
mammalian organs proceed to establish their mass through
definite periods of cellular proliferation, cellular differentiation, and maintenance of mature differentiated
cells. The work reviewed here demonstrates that both brain
and adipose tissue follow this pattern during normal growth,
although the timing of each phase is tissue specific. Once
the adult mass, measured as number of cells is established,
further numerical change cannot be effected by nutritional
means. It is apparent that the nature and quantity of the
nutrients partaken by the young organism plays a definitive
role in defining brain and adipose tissue mass in the mature
organism. Total caloric restriction produced by prenatal
and/or postnatal nutritional manipulation results in the
formation of fewer than normal numbers of cells in both
brain and adipose tissue. The brain is more susceptible to
cell number reduction when the dietary manipulation is begun
in utero because a major portion of brain cell DNA is synthesized before birth. In adipose tissue, it has been recently established that the primary period of hyperplasia
extends until the end of the suckling period in rats. Therefore, adipose tissue is more flexible and responsive to dietary changes introduced postnatally.

Both over and underfeeding during infancy affect fat
cell number. Of further interest is the finding that overfeeding the genetically obese rat leads to a pronounced increase in cell number while underfeeding does not reduce
the cell number, suggesting that dietary effects in the
obese rat are secondary to the genetic regulation of cellular proliferation.

ACKNOWLEDGMENTS

The author wishes to thank Drs. Patricia Johnson, Jo-Anne Brasel, and Myron Winick for the generous use of their illustrations.

References

Bauer, J. (1947). *Am. J. Dig. Diseases* 74, 397.

Bjorntorp, P., and Sjostrom, L. (1971). *Metabolism* 20, 703.

Brasel, J. A., Ehrenkranz, R. A., and Winick, M. (1970). *Develop. Biol.* 23, 424.

Davison, A. N. (1972). *Lipids, Malnutrition, and Developing Brain,* p. 73. Ciba Foundation.

Fish, I., and Winick, M. (1969). *Exp. Neurol.* 25, 534.

Galli, C., White, H. B., and Paoletti, R. (1970). *J. Neurochem.* 17, 347.

Greenwood, M. R. C., and Hirsch, J. (1974). *J. Lipid Res.* 15, 474.

Hellman, B., Taljedal, I. B., and Westman, S. (1962). *Acta Anat.* 55, 286.

Hirsch, J., and Gallian, E. (1968). *J. Lipid Res.* 9, 110.

Hirsch, J., and Han, P. W. (1969). *J. Lipid Res.* 10, 77.

Hirsch, J., and Knittle, J. L. (1970). *Federation Proceedings* 29, 1516.

Hollenberg, C. H., and Vost, A. (1968). *J. Clin. Invest.* 47, 2485.

Johnson, P. R., Stern, J. S., Greenwood, M. R. C., Zucker, L. M., and Hirsch, J. (1973). *J. Nutr.* 103, 738.

Johnson, P. R., Zucker, L. M., Cruce, J. A. F., and Hirsch, J. (1971). *J. Lipid Res.* 12, 706.

Knittle, J. L. Personal Communication.

Knittle, J. L., and Hirsch, J. (1968). *J. Clin. Invest.* 47, 2091.

Lemmonier, D. (1972). *J. Clin. Invest.* 51, 2907.

Mayer, J. (1953). *Physiol. Rev.* 33, 472.

Napolitano, L. (1965). "Handbook of Physiology: Adipose Tissue," p. 109. Amer. Physiol. Soc., New York.

McCance, R. A., and Widdowson, E. M. (1962). *Proc. Roy. Soc.* 156, 326.

O'Brien, J. S., and Sampson, E. L. (1965). *J. Lipid Res.* 6, 545.

Rathbone, L. (1965). *Biochem. J.* 97, 629.

Rodbell, M. (1964). *J. Biol. Chem.* 239, 375.

Rosso, P., Hormazbal, J., and Winick, M. (1970). *Amer. J. Clin. Nutr.* 23, 1275.

Sims, E. A. H., Goldman, R. F., Gluck, C. M., Horton, E. S., Kelleher, P. C., and Rowe, D. W. (1968). *Trans. Assoc. Amer. Physicians* 81, 153.

Stern, J. S., Batchelor, B. R., Hollander, N., Cohn, C. K., and Hirsch, J. (1972). *The Lancet* 2, 948.

White, H. B., Galli, C., and Paoletti, R. (1971). *J. Neurochem.* 18, 869.

Widdowson, E., and Shaw, W. T. (1973). *The Lancet* 2, p. 905.

Winick, M. (1970). *Federation Proceedings* 29, 1510.

Winick, M., and Noble, A. (1965). *Develop. Biol.* 12, 451.

Winick, M., and Noble, A. (1966). *J. Nutr.* 89, 300.

The Influence of Environmental
Factors on Lipid Metabolism

A. SAARI CSALLANY, AND ROGER I. BROOKS

In recent years there has been great interest in the
environment. Many new words such as ecology, environment,
photochemical smog, greenhouse effect, etc. have become
part of our vocabulary. We have simultaneously developed
an awareness of environmental problems caused by the advanced technology created to satisfy our increasing demands
for material comforts. With the population explosion and
technological growth, problems of environmental contamination have become increasingly apparent. Electric power
generating capacity in the United States has increased over
twenty-fold from 1920 to date. There are presently over
45,000 registered pesticide formulations on the Federal
Patent Registry. Synthetic chemical production has more
than doubled in the last ten years. Air pollution and lead
contamination have reached alarmingly high levels in our
cities. Mercury contaminates our lakes and marine life.
Pesticide accumulation has reached high levels in many
species of animals. Chlorine levels are high in our water
supplies. These and many other events have led to intense
national concern about environmental health problems. Evidence of the depth of this concern is illustrated by a variety of recent reports calling attention to environmental
health problems; among these are the widely cited Gross
(1962), Tukey (1965), Spilhaus (1966), and Linton (1967)
reports. National concern has led to a major reorganization
of Federal efforts to solve these problems, including the
establishment in 1968 of an entirely new unit within the
United States Department of Health, Education, and Welfare:
the National Institute of Environmental Health Services.

Society's present concern about environmental contamination exists because urbanization and industrialization
have concentrated large numbers of people in relatively
small areas. Concentrations of pollutants emitted from many
of man's activities have accumulated to levels adverse to

human health and sufficient to produce harmful effects on plant and animal life. An entire symposium could be dedicated to the review of the adverse effects of the numerous environmental factors on *all* phases of lipid metabolism. Therefore, emphasis will be concentrated here on only some of the most important environmental factors related to an important part of lipid metabolism, lipid peroxidation.

In vivo lipid peroxidation has been identified as a basic deteriorative reaction in cellular mechanisms of aging processes (Barber and Bernheim, 1967; Packer *et al.*, 1967), in air pollution oxidant damage to cells (Goldstein and Balchum, 1967) and to lung tissue (Thomas *et al.*, 1967), in some phases of atherosclerosis (Hartroft, 1965; Perkins *et al.*, 1965), in chlorinated hydrocarbon hepatoxicity (Recknagel, 1967; Recknagel, 1973; Recknagel, 1971a; Recknagel, 1971b), in ethanol-induced liver injury (DiLuzio, 1973), in oxygen toxicity (Haugaard, 1968), in irradiation damage (Meffert and Reichmann, 1972), and in vitamin E deficiency diseases (Scott, 1970). Increased understanding of lipid peroxidation and its involvement in the processes of membrane and cellular damage may contribute substantially to the betterment of human health. Lipid peroxidation, caused by free radical initiators present in the environment, may be the basis of the chemical deteriorative mechanisms that cause membrane structure damage and thereby lead to accelerated aging processes. Under stress conditions, these chemical deteriorative reactions may possibly be slowed by the use of increased amounts of dietary antioxidants.

Lipid peroxidation, the reaction of oxidative deterioration of polyunsaturated lipids, involves the production of semistable peroxides from free radical intermediates produced by direct reaction of oxygen with unsaturated lipids. The production of free radicals, mainly peroxy radicals (ROO$\cdot$), alkoxy radicals (RO$\cdot$), and hydroxy radicals ($\cdot$OH), during lipid peroxidation leads to subsequent damaging reactions. Free radicals have unpaired electrons which react very energetically and which initiate relatively nonspecific hydrogen abstraction and chemical addition reactions. Free radicals produced during lipid peroxidation are chemically similar to the damaging radical species produced in irradiation (Fetner, 1958; Brinkman and Lamberts, 1958). Based upon measurements of mole of enzyme inactivated per mole of free radical produced, lipid peroxidation is one-tenth as damaging as ionizing radiation (Chio and

Tappel, 1969). Because of the damaging effects produced, lipid peroxidation is considered one of the most deteriorative of the reactions that results in damage to membranous cellular constituents.

The destructive effects of free radicals on biological systems are best known from studies of their reactions with proteins and enzymes. Enzymes and proteins undergo reactions of polymerization, polypeptide chain scission, and chemical changes in amino acids when subjected to lipid peroxidation (Roubal and Tappel, 1966a; Roubal and Tappel, 1966b). The pattern of damage to proteins induced by peroxidizing lipids similar to that observed in radiation damage.

Quantitative studies of enzyme inactivation by lipid peroxidation show that sulfhydryl enzymes are most susceptible to inactivation (Chio and Tappel, 1969). However, oxidation products of polyunsaturated lipids also inactivate nonsulfhydryl enzymes. Ribonuclease A, when reacted with peroxidizing lipids, simultaneously loses enzyme activity while developing fluorescence. When inactivated by reaction with malonaldehyde, ribonuclease has fluorescence and gel filtration patterns similar to those produced when it is inactivated by peroxidizing polyunsaturated lipids. It is postulated that malonaldehyde (an end product of the peroxidation of polyunsaturated fatty acids) is the reactant for the intramolecular and intermolecular cross-linking of enzymes and proteins. A conjugated amine structure, formed between the amino groups ($-NH_2$) of amino acids, peptides, and proteins with malonaldehyde ($OHC-CH_2-CHO$) is thought responsible for the fluorescence produced by cross-linking of proteins and enzymes. Many biologically important amines including RNA, DNA, and phospholipids cross-link with malonaldehyde to form the fluorescent chromophoric Schiff base structure ($RN=CH-CH=CH-NH-R$). These fluorescent compounds are termed lipofuscin (or age) pigments; they are possibly damaging to cells, especially in higher concentrations. These age pigments have been found to deposit in various body tissues, such as brain, heart, lung, spleen, kidney, liver, and reproductive organs (Strehler *et al.*, 1959). The relative ratios of lipofuscin pigment concentrations of various tissues of normal animals have been found by Csallany and co-workers to be: 1 (lung) : 3.2 (liver) : 4.0 (spleen) : 7 (kidney) : 8.2 (heart) : 12.4 (brain) (Csallany, unpublished data).

199

The major site of lipid peroxidative damage within the cell are at biomembranes, especially those of subcellular organelles. Mitochondrial and microsomal membranes contain relatively large amounts of polyunsaturated fatty acids in their phospholipids. These include fatty acids with 2, 4, 5, and 6 double bonds (Witting, 1965). In addition, some of the most powerful catalysts that initiate lipid peroxidation, such as iron and hemeproteins, are in close proximity to these polyunsaturated lipids. Once initiated, free radical lipid peroxidation proceeds by a chain reaction mechanism through the polyunsaturated fatty acids of the phospholipids in a membrane. Each completed cycle of peroxidation produces a fatty acid hydroperoxide. Peroxide decomposition, a hemolytic scission process promoted by metal catalysts, further accelerates lipid peroxidation and produces hydroxy fatty acids. Most of the damage produced in mitochondrial and microsomal membrane lipid peroxidation occurs through free radical chain cross-linking of enzymes and proteins, oxidative chemical modifications of susceptible amino acids of membrane enzymes and proteins, and carbonyl cross-linking reactions with ethanolamine and serine (Tappel, 1973).

Red blood cell membranes are labile to lipid peroxidation because of their high content of polyunsaturated lipids and the fact that they are directly exposed to oxygen (Hochstein, 1966). Lipid peroxidation leads to hemolysis of the red blood cell. The mechanisms of hemolysis are believed to involve both direct damage to membrane lipid structure and inhibition of erythrocyte acetylcholinesterase activity by lipid peroxides (O'Malley et al., 1966).

The integrity of cell structure and function is especially dependent upon the stability of lysosomal membranes. Lysosomal membrane lysis releases a variety of hydrolytic enzymes capable of producing intracellular digestion and catabolism. These enzymes are able to degrade cellular proteins, lipids, carbohydrates, and nucleic acids. Studies of the effects of lipid peroxidation and free radicals on lysosomes show that they undergo lipid peroxidation less rapidly than mitochondrial or microsomal membranes. Lysosomes peroxidize at one-third the rate of mitochondria and one-tenth the rate of microsomes due to the lysosome's lower lipid content. Exposure of lysosomes to peroxidizing linoleate releases lysosomal hydrolytic enzymes such as arylsulfatase, beta-glucuronidase, acid phosphatase, and ribonuclease. Studies have shown a wide variation in the ability of free radical sources to cause lysosomal enzyme release; however, cysteine, glutathione, ascorbic acid, and ionic iron mixtures have all been shown to cause lysosomal membrane rupture and hydrolytic enzyme release (Tappel, 1973).

Some of the most important environmental factors affecting lipid peroxidation include: (1) gaseous oxidant air pollutants (ozone and nitrogen dioxide); (2) chlorinated hydrocarbons; (3) radiation; (4) heavy metals (zinc, copper, and iron); (cytochrome P-450, an iron-containing component of electron transport systems involved in oxidative pathways, also affects lipid peroxidation); and (5) selenium (a vital constituent of the enzyme glutathione peroxidase).

Oxidants are a major component of photochemical air pollution. Two of the principal identified oxidants found in polluted urban air are ozone (O_3) and nitrogen dioxide (NO_2). These two gases possess similar chemical properties in that both are capable of free radical formation; these free radicals are highly oxidizing in nature.

Ozone and nitrogen dioxide are produced in the upper atmosphere by solar radiation, and small concentrations of these gases are transported to the lower atmosphere near the earth's surface. The result is that normal air contains up to 0.02 ppm of NO_2 (Kuiper, 1952) and from 0.01 to 0.04 ppm of ozone (Lunge, 1963). In polluted urban air, these ranges are much higher. The average concentration of NO_2 in the atmosphere over major U.S. cities ranges from 0.03 to 0.06 ppm. The maximum daily average is 0.10 to 0.26 ppm and the maximum average for a five minute period is 0.24 to 0.79 ppm. Typical ranges for ozone in American cities on smog-free days are 0.05 to 0.20 ppm and on smoggy days 0.30 to 0.65 ppm. Maximum values up to 0.90 ppm have been recorded (Stern, 1968).

Ozone is classified as one of the most highly toxic gases. Studies on the physiological toxicity of ozone show that it is highly injurious, even lethal, to laboratory animals in a single exposure of only a few hours duration (Stokinger, 1957). Physiological effects of ozone inhalation range from dryness of the mucous membranes of the mouth, nose, and throat, changes in visual acuity, and headaches to more serious changes such as functional derangements of the lung, pulmonary congestion, and edema (Stern, 1968). Nitrogen dioxide exposure can also produce

201

a variety of responses in humans. As dosages increase, a-
cute effects are expressed as odor perception, followed con-
secutively by nose and eye irritation, pulmonary congestion,
edema, bronchiolitis, pneumonia, and finally death (Lynn
and McMullen, 1966). Chronic effects of continuous exposure are different from those of intermittent exposure. In
general, the effects of continuous exposure to a given concentration of ozone or NO_2 are more severe than those of
intermittent exposures.

Substantial evidence exists to implicate free radicals
as the biochemical mechanism of ozone and nitrogen dioxide-
induced cell damage. Studies on the similarity of the effects of ozone and NO_2 to those of irradiation have been
conducted by Fetner (1958) and Brinkman and Lamberts (1958).
These and other studies have led to the hypothesis that
ozone is radiomimetic and results in free radical formation.
Several theories have arisen explaining how free radicals
develop during exposure to ozone and NO_2. Fetner (1958)
has suggested that free radicals arise from ozone decomposition in aqueous solutions. Stokinger (1965), after review-
ing the evidence demonstrating the marked lability of sulfhydryl containing compounds to ozone, has suggested that
free radicals develop by the reaction of ozone with sulfhydryl groups. Goldstein (1967) has developed a hypothesis
based on the ability of ozone to react with the double
bonds of unsaturated fatty acids. Ozone reacts rapidly with
double bonds to form ozonides. Therefore, because polyunsaturated fatty acids are primary components of the phospholipids of lipoproteins (important in lipid transport and
membrane structure), fatty ozonides may be a primary product
of the attack of ozone in animal tissues. Free radicals
then can develop from these unstable ozonides or peroxide
intermediates and initiate the chain reaction of lipid peroxidation. Roehm et al. (1971) have theorized that NO_2
adds directly to double bonds to form nitroso-free radicals.
Nitroso-free radicals are capable of initiating lipid peroxidation by abstraction of methylene hydrogen radicals. The
alkyl-free radicals can then react with molecular oxygen to
form fatty acid hydroperoxides, thus generating the conven-
tional peroxidation reactions.

Ozone and NO_2 are widely believed to induce both *in
vivo* and *in vitro* lipid peroxidation. Trace quantities of
ozone and NO_2 (1.5 ppm) have both been shown to catalyze
the rapid peroxidation of unsaturated fatty acid films and
aqueous emulsions. Phenolic antioxidants, including

vitamin E, retard the peroxidation, as measured by the thiobarbituric acid (TBA) test and reduced ultraviolet absorbance at 235 nm of conjugated dienoic hydroperoxides. At equivalent concentrations, ozone has been found to induce lipid peroxidation more rapidly than NO_2 and is less effectively inhibited by phenolic antioxidants (Roehm et al., 1971).

Goldstein and Balchum (1967) have shown that lipid peroxidation is involved in ozone-induced cell membrane damage in an in vitro erythrocyte system. Ozone produces increased levels of TBA reactants. (Thiobarbituric acid is predominantly used to measure malonaldehyde, a breakdown product of lipid peroxidation.) Ultraviolet absorption patterns (diene conjugation) characteristic of lipid peroxidation are also found in the extracted erythrocyte lipids.

In vivo studies on rats continuously exposed for 5 or 7 days to ambient ozone concentrations (0.7 to 0.8 ppm) by Chow and Tappel (1972) have shown that ozone exposure significantly raises the concentration of TBA reactants (principally malonaldehyde) produced by lipid peroxidation. Others (Goldstein et al., 1969) have found ultraviolet absorption patterns denoting the presence of diene and triene systems, considered characteristic of peroxidized lipid, in spectrophotometric analyses of extracted lung lipids of mice and rats continuously exposed to ambient ozone concentrations. Thomas et al. (1968) have found similar lung lipid spectra, after exposure of rats to ambient levels of NO_2. These findings support the view that both ozone and NO_2, at concentrations to which a majority of most metropolitan populations are frequently exposed, can cause lipid peroxidation in animal lungs and other tissues.

According to studies conducted by Fletcher and Tappel (1973), dietary alpha-tocopherol acetate exerts a protective effect in rats exposed to ambient levels of ozone and NO_2, as measured by acute toxicity studies, animal weight studies, and TBA reactant concentrations. Recent studies by Csallany and co-workers (unpublished data) show an approximate 20% weight reduction in mice continuously exposed to low levels of NO_2 (0.5 and 1.0 ppm) for 1 1/2 years. Exposure of rats to 10 ppm NO_2 results in reduction of polyunsaturated fatty acids in the lungs of vitamin E depleted animals, according to Roehm et al. (1971). Csallany and co-workers (unpublished data), however, have not found significant changes in the polyunsaturated fatty acid profiles of lung lipids of rats intermittently exposed to 15 ppm of NO_2 (1 hour/day for 5 months). Vitamin E deficiency in rats is associated with a greater susceptibility to lethal levels of O_3. Exposure to sublethal O_3 concentrations produces accelerated decline in serum vitamin E levels (Cardenas and Buckley, 1970). These findings are consistent with the belief that lipid peroxidation is the mechanism of NO_2 and O_3 toxicity. When washed human erythrocyte suspensions are exposed to 40 ppm O_3, the extracted lipids show significant decreases in oleic (17%), linoleic (27%), and arachidonic (38%) acids according to Balchum et al. (1971). Dietary supplementation with 100 mg of dl-alpha-tocopherol acetate/kg diet extends the survival time for rats exposed to 1.0 ppm of O_3. Toxic symptoms are associated with increased arachidonic and palmitic acid levels and decreased oleic and linoleic acid levels in lung tissues (Rohen et al., 1972). Significantly lower concentrations of palmitic acid have been found by Csallany and co-workers (unpublished data) in lung lipids of rats intermittently exposed to 15 ppm of NO_2 (1 hour/day for 5 months). Purified ozonides and hydroperoxides of methyl linoleate cause death when injected intravenously to rats in a dose 0.07 nmole/100 g body weight. No deaths resulted in a 24 hour period after single oral dosages of these compounds at concentrations ten-fold greater than those causing death by the intravenous route. The major effect of these compounds is on the lungs. These become enlarged from edema and accumulation of fluid, and the animals die of lung congestion and injury similar to the effects of ozone toxicity. There is no vitamin E destruction in the lung tissues of animals given lethal dosages of the compounds intravenously, but significant changes occur in fatty acid composition of the lung and the serum lipids. Arachidonic acid increases at the expense of linoleic and oleic acids in these tissues (Cortes and Privett, 1972). Other studies show that NO_2 induces lipid peroxidation in vivo, and subsequently induces lipofuscin (age) pigment formation (Thomas et al., 1968; Csallany, unpublished data). These pigments appear to be metabolic end products of lipid peroxidation; they deposit in the lung, brain, heart, spleen, and other vital tissues. Vitamin E has been found to lower the effect of NO_2-induced lipid peroxidation in several of these tissues (Csallany, 1972).

Exposure of rats to low levels of ozone has been found by Chow et al. (1974) to promote an enzymatic protective mechanism against lipid peroxidation. This protective mechanism involves the enzyme glutathione (GSH) peroxidase. GSH peroxidase may be responsible for the reductive detoxification of lipid peroxides in tissue, thus protecting cellular components from peroxidative damage (Little and O'Brien, 1968). Exposure of rats to low concentrations of ozone (0.2 to 0.75 ppm) continuously for 8 days, or intermittently (8 hours/day) for 7 days, significantly increases the activity of the GSH peroxidase system in lung tissue. Lysozyme activity is significantly increased in the soluble lung fraction and plasma during continuous ozone exposure, but not during intermittent ozone exposure.

Recent studies by Csallany and co-workers (unpublished data) have shown that continuous exposure of mice to low levels of NO_2 (0.5 ppm and 1.0 ppm) for 1 1/2 years did not significantly increase GSH peroxidase activity in whole blood. Chow et al. (1974) have exposed rats to NO_2 (1.0 to 6.2 ppm) for 4 days and have found the activities of GSH reductase and glucose-6-phosphate dehydrogenase are significantly increased. However, there is no significant increase in GSH peroxidase activity or lysozyme activity during NO_2 exposure. From these results, they suggest that the mechanism of action of NO_2 must be different from that of ozone.

Nitrogen dioxide and ozone, when present at concentrations existing daily in most metropolitan areas, have thus been shown capable of inducing free radical in vivo and in vitro lipid peroxidation. The effects of ozone and NO_2 exposure appear to be similar to those produced by irradiation, although their exact mechanisms of action have not yet been determined. Phenolic antioxidants, especially vitamin E, have been shown to exert a protective inhibitory effect against lipid peroxidation and its subsequent deteriorative action. An enzymic protective mechanism (the glutathione peroxidase-reductase system) has also been found to protect cellular components from gaseous oxidant-induced lipid peroxidation.

A. CHLORINATED HYDROCARBONS

Chlorinated hydrocarbons have been shown to actively induce lipid peroxidation, both in vivo and in vitro. They have been shown to produce hepatoxicity as evidenced by fatty infiltration, liver triglyceride accumulation, hepatic necrosis, and lethality (DiLuzio, 1973).

Carbon tetrachloride is one of the most extensively studied chlorinated hydrocarbons. In carbon tetrachloride poisoning, rat liver microsomal and mitochondrial preparations both produce lipid peroxidation, although it proceeds much more rapidly in liver microsomes than in mitochondria. In these preparations, malonaldehyde is produced, the concentrations of polyunsaturated fatty acids are decreased, and conjugated dienes appear. Srinvasan and Recknagel (1973) have found that oral administration of carbon tetrachloride to rats induces rapid lipid peroxidation of liver and kidney endoplasmic reticulum, as evidenced by the appearance of conjugated dienes. Recknagel and Ghoshal (1966) have proposed a mechanism for CCl_4 toxicity in which free radicals, arising from CCl_4 cleavage, attack the methylene bridges of the unsaturated fatty acid side chains of complex structural lipids found in the endoplasmic reticulum. These free radicals set off autocatalytic chains of peroxidative lipid decomposition. Loss of physiological and biochemical properties of the endoplasmic reticulum then follows, eventually leading to all the previously mentioned pathological consequences of CCl_4 poisoning.

For years it has been known that d-alpha-tocopherol can protect rats from the lethal effects of CCl_4 (Hove, 1948). Antioxidant protection implies that the reaction of the liver to CCl_4 involves destructive lipid peroxidation. Recknagel and Ghoshal's (1966) suggested mechanism that CCl_4 is hemolytically cleaved in the liver to yield a trichloro-methyl free radical ($CCl_3\cdot$) and a monoatomic chlorine-free radical ($Cl\cdot$) which initiate autocatalytic destructive lipid peroxidation of microsomal lipids, is consistent with these findings. The degenerated complex lipids exhibit the characteristic 233 nm absorption of diene conjugation. Ethylene diamine tetracetic acid (EDTA), but not ascorbic acid, prevents the peroxidation of microsomal lipids *in vitro* and the consequent appearance of diene conjugation.

A correlation has been found between the rate of lipid peroxidation and the conversion of cytochrome P-450 to inactive cytochrome P-420 in rats orally administered CCl_4. The endoplasmic cytochrome P-450 content decreased 30-40% within 3 hours after CCl_4 administration (Reiner *et al.*, 1973). EDTA and glutathione inhibit lipid peroxidation in this system and cause the cytochrome P-450 concentrations to remain at control levels.

Studies with hepatic microsomal preparations from rats with CCl_4-induced cirrhosis have shown peroxidative destruction of microsomal phospholipid as evidenced by decreased membranous hydrophobicity and conversion of cytochrome P-450 to inactive cytochrome P-420 (Tsyrlov et al., 1972).

Carbon tetrachloride has also been shown to induce lipid peroxidation in rat adrenals (Castro et al., 1972). Both mitochondrial and microsomal lipids are peroxidized, although there is less damage in mitochondrial lipids. In addition, cytochrome P-450 destruction occurs in the microsomal portion and adrenal lysosomal permeability is increased.

Glutathione has been shown to inhibit CCl_4-induced lipid peroxidation (Reiner et al., 1973). Sodium diethyl-dithiocarbamate has also been found to protect against CCl_4-induced lipid peroxidation (Lutz et al., 1973). Other inhibitors of CCl_4-induced lipid peroxidation include heterocyclic mercaptocompounds (Rauen et al., 1973). The peroxidation in rat liver endoplasmic reticular phospholipid membrane by CCl_4 is strongly inhibited by intraperitoneal treatment with 3,5-dimercapto-isothiozole-4-carboxamide (most effective), 1,3,4-thiadiazole-2,5-dithiol, 1,2,3-trizole-3-thiol, DL-3-aminotetrahydro-2-thiophenone, and L-cysteine (Rauen et al., 1973). A study by McLean and McLean (1966) has shown that protein depleted rats are resistant to the lethal effects and to the liver-damaging effects of CCl_4. DDT and phenobarbitone destroy this resistance. Phenobarbital has been shown to promote CCl_4-induced lipid peroxidation in mice (Riely and Cohen, 1974) and in beagle dogs (Litterst et al., 1973).

Other chlorinated hydrocarbons have been found to produce hepatoxicity and liver dysfunction. These include chloroform, 1,1,2-trichloroethane, trichloroethylene, and 1,1,1-trichloroethane (Traiger and Plaa, 1974). Hepatic microsomal lipid peroxidation has also been found to be induced by other chlorinated hydrocarbons. Chloroform and halothane, two chlorinated hydrocarbons used in inhalation anaesthetics, have been found to induce in vivo lipid peroxidation in rat liver microsomal lipids (Brown, 1972). Pretreatment with phenobarbital also enhances lipid peroxidation in the rat liver microsomal lipids of these systems.

207

Ethanol administration has been demonstrated to increase *in vivo* and *in vitro* peroxidation of hepatic lipids just as chlorinated hydrocarbons have (DiLuzio and Hartman, 1967). It is believed that ethanol induces free radical chain reactions in the liver, and that antioxidants act as inhibitors of peroxidative lipid degeneration. Studies by DiLuzio (1973) have shown that N,N'-diphenyl-p-phenylenediamine (DPPD), a lipid antioxidant, significantly inhibits ethanol-induced peroxidation in the liver. These studies show that antioxidants are more effective in preventing fibrotic and cirrhotic alterations and in maintaining liver function than in inhibiting the development of fatty liver.

DiLuzio and co-workers (1973) have found that the effects of ethanol and CCl_4-induced hepatic lipid peroxidation are very similar. Diene conjugation absorption studies (200-340 nm) of rat liver microsomal and mitochondrial lipids have been conducted at various intervals after ethanol and CCl_4 administration. The data obtained from the CCl_4 experiments confirm the observations of Recknagel and Ghoshal (1966) of the presence of conjugated dienes in the microsomal fraction of CCl_4-treated rats. However, the microsomal lipid fraction of ethanol-treated rats does not exhibit diene conjugation (233 nm). The mitochondrial lipid fraction of ethanol-treated rats shows the presence of enhanced absorption at 233 nm, while the mitochondrial lipid fraction of CCl_4-treated animals does not exhibit enhanced absorption. These studies suggested the possibility that comparable effects of lipid peroxidation, with a differential subcellular localization, occur in CCl_4 and ethanol-treated rats. To further investigate these findings, DiLuzio and Hartman (1967) have determined the lipid-soluble antioxidants in the microsomal and mitochondrial fractions of CCl_4 and ethanol-treated rats. Antioxidant concentrations of mitochondria are significantly reduced in the ethanol-treated group. The microsomal lipid-soluble antioxidant concentration is not significantly different than the control value in the ethanol-treated group. In contrast to the results with ethanol, CCl_4 administration results in reduction in the concentration of microsomal lipid-soluble antioxidants, but does not result in mitochondrial lipid-soluble antioxidant reduction. Thus, DiLuzio and co-workers conclude that ethanol-induced conjugated diene formation is mitochondrial in nature, while CCl_4-induced conjugated diene formation is microsomal. DiLuzio (1973) has also proposed a hypothesis for the induction of liver peroxidative injury by hepatotoxic agents such as ethanol and CCl_4 and for the

possible sites of the inhibitory action of antioxidants
(Fig. 1). Inhibitory action occurs at the A[*] sites by
either prevention of oxidative degradation leading to the
formation of lipoperoxides, hydroperoxides, or polymers, or
by termination of the chain reaction induced by free radicals. Inhibition at site B[*] occurs by decomposition of
peroxides to produce inactive products.

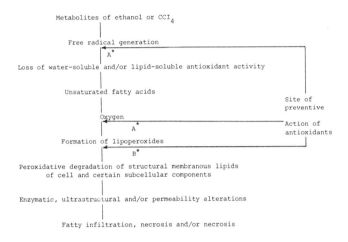

Metabolites of ethanol or CCl_4

Free radical generation

A[*]

Loss of water-soluble and/or lipid-soluble antioxidant activity

Unsaturated fatty acids

Oxygen

A[*]

Formation of lipoperoxides

B[*]

Peroxidative degradation of structural membranous lipids
of cell and certain subcellular components

Enzymatic, ultrastructural and/or permeability alterations

Fatty infiltration, necrosis and/or necrosis

Site of
preventive
Action of
antioxidants

Fig. 1. Proposed hypothesis of liver injury and antioxidant inhibitory sites.

Fig. 1. From DiLuzio (1973).

Although ethanol is not an environmental factor in
lipid peroxidation, its peroxidative mechanism is closely
related to the mechanism of carbon tetrachloride-induced
lipid peroxidation. Several workers have proposed possible
explanations for the mechanism by which ethanol stimulates
the lipoperoxidation of liver preparations and liver tissue. As previously stated, DiLuzio and Hartman (1973) have
found that acute ethanol intoxication causes a decrease in
the lipid-soluble antioxidant concentration in liver
mitochondria. Lieber and DeCarli (1970) have found enhanced NADPH oxidase activity in liver microsomes of rats
fed ethanol for several days. Takada et al. (1970) have
reported finding lowered contents of reduced glutathione

(CSH) in whole liver of ethanol-treated rats. Cherrick and Leevy (1965) have found changes in the redox state of the liver cells occurring as a consequence of ethanol metabolism (changes in the NAD/NADH ratio and increases in the reduced pyridine coenzymes). All of these phenomena could affect hepatic lipid peroxidation.

Chlorinated hydrocarbons (especially CCl_4) and ethanol have thus been shown to induce both *in vivo* and *in vitro* lipid peroxidation. Although the effects of CCl_4 and ethanol-induced lipid peroxidation are similar, peroxidation occurs in different subcellular locales. CCl_4-induced peroxidation occurs mainly in microsomal lipids while ethanol-induced peroxidation occurs in mitochondrial lipids. Antioxidants, alpha-tocopherol and DPPD, have been shown to effectively inhibit lipid peroxidation induced by both compounds. Several mechanisms of CCl_4 and ethanol-induced lipid peroxidation have been proposed, but the exact mechanism has not yet been elucidated.

B. RADIATION

Free radicals can be produced by the absorption of light or high energy radiation (Burr, 1968). X-ray, gamma ray, and ultraviolet radiation have each been shown to produce increased lipid peroxidation. Ahlers *et al.* (1973) have found that continuous gamma irradiation (60 R./day for 25 days) significantly increases the concentration of lipid peroxides in liver and kidney tissues. Dancewicz (1972) has irradiated rats with 750 R. and has found increased concentrations of lipid peroxides in liver and spleen subcellular fractions. Irradiation also lowers the sulf-hydryl (-SH) content of these fractions and affects the distribution of several enzymes within the cell's subcellular components. Roshchupkin *et al.* (1973) have found ultraviolet radiation-induced photo-oxidation of mitochondrial lipids to produce lipid peroxides and cause inactivation of the physiological functions of the mitochondria. X-ray irradiation has been found to produce increased hydrolytic enzyme activity in liver perfusates and in lysosomal and mitochondrial fractions (Deby, 1971). Lipid peroxidation products (lipid peroxides, hydroperoxides, and malonaldehyde) have been found to increase in rat liver, spleen, heart, and kidney following whole body X-ray irradiation (Aono *et al.*, 1972). Injection of polyunsaturated fatty acid esters into rats, following X-ray irradiation

(750 R.), results in an 8-fold increase in lipid peroxide
concentration in exposed animals versus the nonexposed
controls (Deby, 1971).

Radiation-induced *in vitro* lipid peroxidation has also
been investigated. Irradiation of mouse liver homogenates
with 500-2,000 R. results in increased concentrations of
lipid peroxidation products. Similar results have been
obtained using heart, spleen, and kidney homogenates (Dawes
and Wills, 1972).

Ascorbic acid and ferrous ions have both been shown to
promote lipid peroxidation in liver homogenates of irradiated rats (Aono *et al.*, 1972). Beta-mercaptoethylamine
(Goncharenko, 1971), platonin (a photosensitive dye) (Aono
et al., 1972), dietary butylated hydroxy toluene (BHT)
(Dawes and Wills, 1972), and dietary alpha-tocopherol (Dawes
and Wills, 1972) have each been shown to inhibit radiation-
induced lipid peroxidation.

Studies by Meffert and Reichmann (1972) have shown the
effect of ultraviolet radiation on lipid peroxidation of
human skin surfaces. The concentration of lipid peroxides
on the skin's surface has been found to increase with increasing radiation dosage. However, the malonaldehyde concentration and the fatty acid profiles remain unchanged.

C. HEAVY METALS

Relatively little is known about the effects of heavy
metals upon the processes of lipid peroxidation. The work
reported here has been concentrated on the effects of zinc
and iron salts. These two metals appear to produce opposite
effects upon lipid peroxidation; zinc acts as an inhibitor
and iron as a promoter of lipid peroxidation.

Experiments performed by Chvapil *et al.* (1974) have
demonstrated that dietary zinc can inhibit lipid peroxidation in rat liver tissue and red blood cells. High concentrations of dietary zinc (1,000 ppm) produce significant
decreases in the induction and rate of formation of malonaldehyde as compared to low concentrations (40 ppm) and
control levels. Zinc also produces a specific effect upon
the fatty acid profiles of rat liver tissues. The
arachidonic acid content of the livers of rats being fed a
low zinc diet (40 ppm) is significantly decreased after

lipid peroxidation; such decreases in arachidonic acid following lipid peroxidation are not observed in animals fed the high zinc diet (1,000 ppm).

Chvapil *et al.* (1973) have also shown that CCl_4-induced rat liver injury is substantially reduced by zinc treatment. In rats treated with CCl_4, a significant increase in microsomal and mitochondrial malonaldehyde content occurred. After intragastric zinc acetate administration (1,000 ppm) to rats receiving CCl_4, the content of malonaldehyde in the hepatic microsomal and mitochondrial fractions is significantly reduced. These results agree in many respects with the report of Saldeen (1969), who has used a histological method to evaluate liver lesion formation. He has also demonstrated the protective action of zinc against CCl_4-induced liver damage.

Bidlack and Tappel (1972) have proposed that the possible mechanism of stabilization of biomembranes by dietary zinc is related to lipid peroxidation, specifically to the NADPH oxidation-related formation of free radicals which initiate the peroxidation reactions. NADPH oxidase (cytochrome C reductase), involved in lipid peroxidation, requires the presence of NADPH, iron (Fe^{+2} or Fe^{+3}), and oxygen and is inhibited by the presence of zinc (Zn^{+2}), calcium (Ca^{+2}), and cobalt (Co^{+2}). The inhibitory effect of zinc on lipid peroxidation is probably due to its interaction at this point in the lipid peroxidation process to prevent formation of free radicals.

Chvapil *et al.* (1974) have also found that dietary zinc cannot inhibit lipid peroxidation in tissues other than liver and red blood cells. Zinc produces no similar peroxidation inhibition in brain, kidney, lung, and testes. This probably is due to each tissue's capacity to retain zinc in proportion to dietary zinc intake. Liver and red blood cells show significant increases in zinc content with increased dietary zinc intake; the other tissues do not show such an increase.

It is well known that many transition metals can catalyze autoxidative processes (Pryor, 1966). For example, copper can cause autoxidative rancidity in dairy products, and iron catalyzes the decomposition of hydroperoxides as follows.

$$Fe^{+2} + ROOH \longrightarrow Fe^{+3} + RO \cdot + OH^-$$

$$\underline{Fe^{+3} + ROOH \longrightarrow Fe^{+2} + ROO \cdot + H^+}$$

Sum: $\qquad 2ROOH \longrightarrow RO \cdot + ROO \cdot + H_2O$

Lipid peroxidation is known to be catalyzed by hemoglobin, iron protoporphyrin, and iron salts. It appears that this type of catalysis is very important in peroxidations that occur in biological systems.

The involvement of iron and copper in lipid peroxidation has been demonstrated by several workers. Fujita (1972) has studied the interrelationships among lipid peroxidation, lipid composition, and cytochrome oxidase activity in rat liver mitochondria. Metal ions (Fe^{+2}, Fe^{+3}, and Cu^{+2}) have been found to catalyze lipid peroxidation by increasing the formation of lipid peroxides. These ions also decrease cytochrome oxidase activity and the unsaturated fatty acid content of the mitochondrial membrane. Total sulfhydryl content of liver microsomes and of the soluble fraction are also decreased by ferrous iron (Fujita, 1974).

Cheremisine *et al.* (1972) have found iron to increase *in vitro* lipid peroxidation. Ferrous sulfate (10^{-4} to 10^{-6} M) increased hydroperoxide concentrations in oxidized oleic acid and in rat liver mitochondrial suspensions. This is accompanied by oxidation of Fe^{+2} to Fe^{+3}, oxygen uptake, and a chemilluminescent flash.

Wills (1972) has shown nonheme iron to increase the formation of lipid peroxides in rat liver microsomes. Rats injected with iron show increased levels of nonheme and total iron in liver microsomal fractions. Liver microsomes from these animals show a 14% increase in lipid peroxide concentration. This results in a partial disintegration of endoplasmic reticulum membranes and loss of various membrane-related functions such as oxidative demethylation. Wills postulates that a small portion of the injected iron is converted into an electron transport component which increases the rate of NADPH-induced lipid peroxidation.

The participation of iron in lipid peroxidation, through a NADPH-induced lipid peroxidation system, was first described by Hochstein and Ernster (1963). The requirements of the NADPH oxidase system include NADPH, iron (Fe^{+2} or

213

Fe^{+3}), and oxygen. Bidlack and Tappel's (1972) proposed system of iron's participation in lipid peroxidation is shown in Fig. 2.

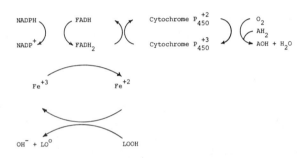

Fig. 2. Proposed mechanism of NADPH-induced lipid peroxidation.

Fig. 2. From Bidlack and Tappel (1972).

It involves catalysis of the reduction of ferric iron to ferrous iron and the subsequent cleavage of hydroperoxides, resulting from Fe^{+2} to Fe^{+3} oxidations, to produce free radical initiators of the peroxidation process.

Wills (1972) and Fujita (1972) have both shown that administration of ascorbic acid along with iron greatly increases lipid peroxidation as compared to iron alone. Wills has reported that rats injected with iron plus ascorbic acid show a 74% increase in hepatic microsomal lipid peroxidation as compared to a 14% increase for iron administration only. It is thought that ascorbate can utilize iron in the normally stored form of ferritin to catalyze lipid peroxidation. This would seem logical in view of the proposed mechanism of Bidlack and Tappel, since ascorbate could act as a reducing agent to maintain the iron in a ferrous state. This would promote enhanced cleavage of hydroperoxides to produce additional free radical lipid peroxidation initiators.

Iron has also been found to be a vital component of cytochrome P-450, an oxidase involved in the electron transfer system associated with lipid peroxidation (DeMatteis and Sparks, 1973). Cytochrome P-450 is the terminal oxidase of the electron transport system involved in the metabolism of a wide variety of substrates such as insecticides, steroids, drugs, and chemical carcinogens. It has also been connected with lipid peroxidation because of its peroxidase activity.

In an *in vitro* system consisting of rat liver microsomes and NADPH studied by Levin *et al.* (1973), lipid peroxidation has been observed along with an accompanying loss of cytochrome P-450. This loss of cytochrome P-450 is the result of a breakdown of cytochrome P-450 heme as shown by radioactive labeling studies. Inhibitors of lipid peroxidation, such as EDTA, α-tocopherol, $MnCl_2$, or $CoCl_2$, prevent the loss of cytochrome P-450, demonstrating a direct relationship between lipid peroxidation and cytochrome P-450 heme breakdown, microsomal polyunsaturated fatty acid loss, and formation of malonaldehyde.

Other studies conducted by Schacter *et al.* (1972) have found that the stimulation of rat liver microsomal lipid peroxidation by ADP and $FeCl_3$ is associated with the rapid degradation of cytochrome P-450 heme and a simultaneous evolution of carbon monoxide. Heme degradation is believed to occur by the fission of one methylene bridge in the tetrapyrrole ring.

Several lines of evidence have also been produced to implicate cytochrome P-450 as the microsomal peroxidase responsible for the rapid decomposition of lipid peroxides by liver microsomes. Cytochrome P-450 can be converted by a wide variety of treatments to a specially modified form called cytochrome P-420. Cytochrome P-420 is inactive as a terminal oxidase in the electron transport chain, but has far greater peroxidase activity than cytochrome P-450. The conversion of cytochrome P-450 to cytochrome P-420 is accompanied by alterations in the hydrophobic environment around the heme moiety and by changes in conformation of the protein component which result in increased exposure of the heme group to the environment and make the protein-bound iron readily available for catalyzing lipid peroxide decomposition. Figure 3 briefly summarizes the peroxidase activity of cytochrome P-450 as proposed by Hrycay and O'Brien (1971).

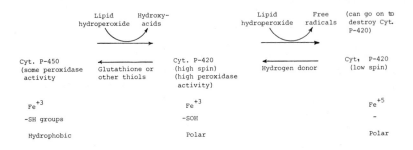

Fig. 3. From Hrycay and O'Brien (1971).

Recent Russian studies by Raikhman and Annaev (1971) have shown that free radicals produced during the conversion of cytochrome P-420 (high spin) to cytochrome P-420 (low spin) may be formed by a two-step process. The first step consists of the oxidation of the heme moiety of cytochrome P-420. This is followed by formation of radical forms of aromatic amino acid residues from the protein component of the cytochrome, as a result of the oxidation of these residues by the oxygen activated on the heme moiety of cytochrome.

Zinc and iron have thus been shown to produce opposite effects upon lipid peroxidation. Dietary zinc inhibits *in vivo* lipid peroxidation in rat liver tissue and red blood cells; however, it does not produce inhibition in other tissues. This is believed due to each tissue's capacity to retain dietary zinc. Copper and iron have each been shown to promote *in vivo* lipid peroxidation by increasing peroxide formation and decreasing sulfhydryl content. Iron is believed to participate in lipid peroxidation through an NADPH-induced system, oxidizing Fe^{+2} to Fe^{+3} to produce peroxide cleavage. Ascorbic acid has been shown to act synergistically with iron to promote increased lipid peroxidation. Iron has also been shown to be a vital component of cytochrome P-450, a terminal oxidase in steroid metabolism, shown to possess peroxidase activity. Cytochrome P-450 reduces lipid peroxides to hydroxy fatty acids while being oxidized to metabolically inactive cytochrome P-420.

D. SELENIUM (AND GLUTATHIONE PEROXIDASE)

Selenium is an essential micronutrient for animals and bacteria. Low dietary levels have been shown to prevent death from deficiency in a variety of species. High dietary levels are extremely toxic and may possibly be carcinogenic. A nutritional requirement for selenium (Se) has been demonstrated by its ability to prevent dietary liver necrosis in vitamin E-deficient rats (Schwartz and Foltz, 1957). Dietary selenium has also been shown to be effective in preventing exudative diathesis in chicks (Scott, 1962), white muscle disease in lambs (Muth and Schubert, 1958), and calves (Muth et al., 1961), and liver necrosis in pigs (Eggert et al., 1957).

Dietary selenium has been found to prevent oxidative damage to rat erythrocytes incubated in vitro, as evidenced by decreased hemolysis and decreased hemoglobin oxidation (Rotruck et al., 1971). Other investigators have found that dietary selenium acts synergistically with vitamin E to alleviate peroxidative stress. These results lead to the hypothesis that selenium may play a role in the protection of animal tissues from damage initiated by lipid peroxidation. This enzymatic protective system, composed of glutathione peroxidase, glutathione reductase, and glucose-6-phosphate dehydrogenase, decomposes lipid peroxides and reduces them to the corresponding hydroxy acids (Little and O'Brien, 1968; Christoffersen, 1969). It thus appears to be an important mechanism to detoxify peroxides.

Evidence implicating selenium as a vital part of the enzyme, glutathione peroxidase, has been found by Rotruck et al. (1973). They have shown that glutathione (GSH) fails to protect selenium-deficient rats from H_2O_2-induced hemoglobin oxidation and erythrocyte hemolysis. Since the hemolysates are devoid of GSH peroxidase activity, it is postulated that selenium is a necessary constituent of the enzyme. They also have shown that ^{75}Se in rat tissue hemolysates coelutes with GSH peroxidase upon chromatographic purification. Subsequent studies have shown that GSH peroxidase, purified to homogeneity, from ovine erythrocytes contains 4 moles of selenium per mole of GSH peroxidase (Flohe *et al.*, 1973). Recent studies conducted by Chow and Tappel (1974) and Hafeman *et al.* (1974) with rat tissues and by Omaye and Tappel (1974) with chick tissues have shown that selenium is essential for the activity of GSH peroxidase and that GSH peroxidase activity increases with increasing dietary levels of selenium.

Work done by Chow and Tappel (1972) has shown the GSH peroxidase-GSH reductase system to be involved in an *in vivo* protective system against lipid peroxidation damage to cellular components. Exposure of rats to ozone causes increased lipid peroxidation, as measured by elevated concentrations of TBA reactants (primarily malonaldehyde). Simultaneous with this increase, elevated levels of GSH peroxidase, GSH reductase, and glucose-6-phosphate dehydrogenase are observed. It is postulated that these elevated enzyme levels act as a compensatory mechanism against increased lipid peroxidation. A visual summary of the reaction mechanism involved is shown in Fig. 4.

Glutathione peroxidase catalyzes the conversion of GSH to GSSG while simultaneously reducing fatty acid hydroperoxides to hydroxy fatty acids. It acts to eliminate toxic fatty acid hydroperoxides that could produce peroxidative damage and converts them to hydroxy fatty acids that can be metabolized by beta-oxidation. The observed elevated levels of GSH reductase are explained by the need for regeneration of GSH from GSSG. GSH reductase insures that reduced gluthathione is recycled within the system. The observed elevation in the level of glucose-6-phosphate dehydrogenase is logical since there is an increased need for NADPH reducing power. The same protective system may also function against lipid peroxidation induced by NO_2 exposure, hyperoxia, CCl_4, ethanol, and other free radical inducing agents.

Increased activity of GSH peroxidase in animal tissues can be produced by an increased rate of enzyme synthesis or a decreased rate of enzyme degradation, or a combination of both. Results obtained by Chow and Tappel (1974) support the decreased enzyme degradation alternative. Injection of rats with puromycin, a protein synthesis inhibitor, and actinomycin D, a RNA synthesis inhibitor, fail to suppress the increase of GSH peroxidase activity in tissues during

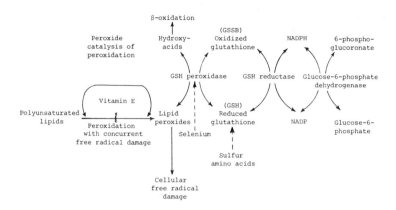

Fig. 4. A summary of the reaction mechanisms involved in the action of the glutathione peroxides - reductase system.

Fig. 4. From Chow and Tappel (1974).

selenium supplementation.

Thus, the GSH peroxidase-reductase system appears to act as an *in vivo* mechanism for the detoxification of lipid hydroperoxides. Lipid hydroperoxides are reduced to hydroxy fatty acids at the expense of GSH which is oxidized to GSSG by GSH peroxidase. GSH reductase then regenerates GSSG back into GSH by employing NADPH for reducing power. In this way, the GSH peroxidase-reductase system functions to prevent the accumulation of lipid hydroperoxides in animal tissues which could lead to peroxidative damage.

References

Ahlers, I., Ahlersova, E., Sedlakova, A., and Praslicka, M. (1973). *Radiobiologiya* 13, 116.

Aono, K., Tanabe, M., Iida, S., Kumada, Y., Utsumi, K., and Yamamoto, M. (1972). *Kanko Shikiso* 82, 13.

Balchum, O. J., O'Brien, J. S., and Goldstein, B. D. (1971). *Arch. Environ. Health* 22, 32.

Barber, A. A., and Bernheim, F. (1967). *In* "Advances in Gerontological Research" (B. L. Strehler, ed.), p. 355, v. 2. Academic Press, New York.

Bidlack, W. R., and Tappel, A. L. (1972). *Lipids* 7, 564.

Brinkman, R., and Lamberts, H. B. (1958). *Nature* 181, 1202.

Brown, B. R., Jr. (1972). *Anesthesiology* 36, 458.

Burr, J. G. (1968). *Advan. Photochem.* 6, 193.

Cardenas, R., and Buckley, R. D. (1970). *Science* 169, 605.

Castro, J. A., Diaz Gomes, M. I., DeFerreyra, E. C., DeCastro, C. R., D'Acosta, N., and DeFeros, O. M. (1972). *Biochem. Biophys. Res. Commun.* 47, 315.

Cheremisine, Z. P., Olenev, V. I., and Valdimirov, Y. A. (1972). *Biofizika* 17, 605.

Cherrick, G. R., and Leevy, C. M. (1965). *Biochem. Biophys. Acta* 107, 29.

Chio, K. S., and Tappel, A. L. (1969). *Biochem.* 8, 2827.

Chow, C. K., and Tappel, A. L. (1972). *Lipids* 7, 518.

Chow, C. K., and Tappel, A. L. (1974). *J. Nutr.* 104, 444.

Chow, C. K., Dillard, C. J., and Tappel, A. L. (1974). *Environ. Res.* 7, 311.

Christoffersen, B. O. (1969). *Biochem. Biophys. Acta* 176, 463.

Cortes, R., and Privett, O. S. (1972). *Lipids* 7, 715.

Csallany, A. S. Unpublished Data.

Csallany, A. S. (1972). *Ill. Res.* 14, 3.

Chvapil, M., Ryan, J. N., Elias, S. L., and Peng, Y. M. (1973). *Exp. Mol. Pathol.* 19, 186.

Chvapil, M., Peng, Y. M., Aronson, A. L., and Zukoski, C. (1974). *J. Nutr.* 104, 434.

Dancewicz, A. M. (1972). "Pervichnye Nachal'nye Protsessy Biol. Deistviye Radiats," p. 195. Dokl. Mezhdunar Simp., 2nd.

Dawes, E. A., and Wills, E. D. (1972). *Int. J. Radiat. Biol.* 22, 23.

Deby, C. (1971). *Arch. Int. Physiol. Biochim.* 79, 626.

DeMatteis, F., and Sparks, R. G. (1973). *FEBS Letters* 29, 141.

DiLuzio, N. R. (1973). *Federation Proceedings* 32, 1875.

DiLuzio, N. R., and Hartman, A. D. (1967). *Federation Proceedings* 26, 1436.

Eggert, R. O., Patterson, E., Akers, W. T., and Stokstad, E. L. R. (1957). *J. Anim. Sci.* 16, 1037.

Fetner, B. H. (1958). *Nature* 181, 504.

Fletcher, B. L., and Tappel, A. L. (1973). *Environ. Res.* 6, 165.

Flohe, L., Gunzler, W. A., and Schock, H. H. (1973). *FEBS Letters* 32, 132.

Fujita, T. (1972). *Yakugaka Zasshi* 92, 250.

Fujita, T. (1974). *Yakugaka Zasshi* 94, 215.

Goldstein, B. D., and Balchum, O. J. (1967). *Proc. Soc. Exptl. Biol. Med.* 126, 356.

Goldstein, B. D., Lodi, C., Collinson, M. T., and Balchum, O. J. (1969). *Arch. Environ. Health* 18, 631.

Goncharenko, E. N. (1971). *Radiobiologiya* 11, 811.

Gross, P. M. (1962). Chairman, Report of the Committee on Environmental Health Problems. Prepared for the Surgeon General, Public Health Service, U.S. Department of Health, Education, and Welfare, 288 pages. U.S. Government Printing Office, Washington, D.C.

Hafeman, D. G., Sunde, R. A., and Hoekstra, W. G. (1974). *J. Nutr.* 104, 580.

Hartroft, W. S. (1965). *In* "Metabolism of Lipids as Related to Atherosclerosis" (F. A. Kummerow, ed.), p. 18. Charles C. Thomas Publishing Company, Springfield, Illinois.

Haugaard, N. (1968). *Physiological Rev.* 48, 331.

Hochstein, P. (1966). *In* "Proceedings of the 3rd International Conference on Hyperbaric Medicine" (I. W. Brown, Jr. and B. G. Cox, eds.), p. 61. National Academy of Sciences, National Research Council, Washington, D.C.

Hochstein, P., and Ernster, L. (1963). *Biochem. Biophys. Res. Commun.* 12, 388.

Hove, E. L. (1948). *Arch. Biochem.* 7, 467.

Hrycay, E. G., and O'Brien, P. J. (1971). *Arch. Biochem. Biophys.* 147, 14.

Kocmierska-Grodzka, D. (1972). *Strahlentherapie* 143, 705.

Kuiper, G. P. (1952). *In* "The Atmospheres of the Earth and Planets," 2nd edition. University of Chicago Press, Chicago.

Levin, W., Lu, A. Y. H., Jacobson, M., and Kurtzman, R. (1973). *Arch. Biochem. Biophys.* 158, 812.

Lieber, C. S., and DeCarli, L. M. (1970). *Science* 170, 78.

Linton, R. M. (1967). Chairman, A Strategy for a Liveable Environment. Report of a Task Force on Environmental Health and Related Problems. Prepared for the Secretary, U.S. Department of Health, Education, and Welfare, 90 pages. U.S. Government Printing Office, Washington, D.C.

Litterst, C. L., Farber, T. M., and Van Loon, E. J.
    (1973). *Toxicol. Appl. Pharmacol.* 25, 354.
Little, C., and O'Brien, P. J. (1968). *Biochem. Biophys.
    Res. Commun.* 31, 145.
Lunge, C. E. (1963). *In* "Air Chemistry and Radioactivity."
    Academic Press, New York.
Lutz, L. M., Glende, E. A., Jr., and Recknagel, R. O.
    (1973). *Biochem. Pharmacol.* 22, 1729.
Lynn, A. D., and McMullen, T. B. (1966). *J. Air
    Pollution Control Assoc.* 16, 186.
McLean, A. E. M., and McLean, E. K. (1966). *Biochem. J.*
    98, *564.*
Meffert, H., and Reichmann, G. (1972). *Acta Biol. Med.
    Ger.* 28, 667.
Muth, O. H., Schubert, J. R., and Oldfield, J. E. (1961).
    Amer. J. Vet. Res. 22, 466.
Muth, O. H., Schubert, J. R., Oldfield, J. E., and Remmert,
    L. F. (1958). *Science* 128, 1090.
O'Malley, B. W., Mengel, C. E., Meriwether, W. D., and
    Zirkle, L. G., Jr. (1966). *Biochem.* 5, 40.
Omaye, S. T., and Tappel, A. L. (1974). *J. Nutr.* 104,
    747.
Packer, L., Deamer, D. W., and Heath, R. L. (1967). *In*
    "Advances in Gerontological Research" (B. L. Strehler,
    ed.), p. 77, v. 2. Academic Press, New York.
Perkins, E. G., Joh, T. H., and Kummerow, F. A. (1965).
    In "Metabolism of Lipids as Related to Atherosclerosis"
    (F. A. Kummerow, ed.), p. 48. Charles C. Thomas
    Publishing Company, Springfield, Illinois.
Pryor, W. A. (1966). *In* "Free Radicals." McGraw-Hill
    Publishing Company, New York.
Raikhman, L. M., and Annaev, B. (1971). *Biokhimiya* 36,
    263.
Rauen, H. M., Schriewer, H., Tegtbauer, U., and Lasana,
    J. E. (1973). *Arzneim.-Forsch.* 23, 145.
Recknagel, R. O. (1967). *Pharmacological Rev.* 19, 145.
Recknagel, R. O. (1971a). *Exp. Mol. Pathol.* 15, 230.
Recknagel, R. O. (1971b). *J. Lipid Res.* 12, 766.
Recknagel, R. O. (1973). "Liver," p. 150.
Recknagel, R. O., and Ghoshal, A. K. (1966). *Nature* 210,
    1162.
Reiner, O., Athanassopoulos, S., Hellmer, K. H., Murray,
    R. E., and Uehleke, H. (1973). *Arch. Toxicol.* 29,
    219.
Riely, C. A., and Cohen, G. (1974). *Science* 183, 208.

Roehm, J. N., Hadley, J. G., and Menzel, D. B. (1971a).
Arch. Intern. Med. 128, 88.
Roehm, J. N., Hadley, J. G., and Menzel, D. B. (1971b).
Arch. Environ. Health 23, 142.
Rohen, J. F., Hadley, J. G., Menzel, D. B. and Wash, R.
(1972). *Arch. Environ. Health* 24, 237.
Roshchupkin, D. I., Marzoev, A. I., and Vladimirov, Y. A.
(1973). *Biotizika* 18, 83.
Rotruck, J. T., Hoekstra, W. G., and Pope, A. L. (1971).
Nature New Biol. 231, 223.
Rotruck, J. T., Pope, A. L., Ganther, H. E., Swanson, A. B.,
Hafeman, D. G., and Hoekstra, W. G. (1973). *Science*
179, 588.
Roubal, W. T., and Tappel, A. L. (1966a). *Arch. Biochem.*
Biophys. 113, 5.
Roubal, W. T., and Tappel, A. L. (1966b). *Arch. Biochem.*
Biophys. 113, 150.
Saldeen, T. (1969). *Z. Ges. Exp. Med.* 150, 251.
Schacter, B. A., Marver, H. S., and Meyer, U. A. (1972).
Biochem. Biophys. Acta 279, 221
Schwartz, K., and Foltz, C. M. (1957). *J. Amer. Chem.*
Soc. 79, 3292.
Scott, M. L. (1962). *Vitamins Hormones* 20, 621.
Scott, M. L. (1970). "The Fat-Soluble Vitamins" (H. F.
DeLuca and J. W. Suttie, eds.), p. 355. University of
Wisconsin Press, Madison, Wisconsin.
Srinvasan, S., and Recknagel, R. O. (1973). *Exp. Mol.*
Pathol. 18, 214.
Stern, A. C. (1968). *In* "Air Pollution," v. 1, 2nd
edition. Academic Press, New York.
Stokinger, H. E. (1957). *Arch. Ind. Health* 15, 181.
Stokinger, H. E. (1965). *Arch. Environ. Health* 10, 719.
Spilhaus, A. (1966). Chairman, Waste Management Control.
Report of the Committee on Pollution to the Federal
Council for Science and Technology, Publication 1400,
257 pages. National Academy of Sciences, National
Research Council, Washington, D.C.
Strehler, B. L., Mark, D. D., Mildvan, A. S., and Gee,
M. V. (1959). *J. Gerontol.* 14, 430.
Takeda, A., Ikegami, F., Okumura, Y., Hasumura, Y.,
Kanayama, R., and Takeuchi, J. (1970). *Lab. Invest.*
23, 421.
Tappel, A. L. (1973). *Federation Proceedings* 32, 1870.
Thomas, H. V., Mueller, P. K., and Lyman, R. L. (1967).
Science 159, 532.
Thomas, H. V., Mueller, P. K., and Lyman, R. L. (1968).
Science 159, 532.

Traiger, G. J., and Plaa, G. L. (1974). *Arch. Environ. Health* 28, 276.

Tsyrlov, I. B., Mishin, V. M., and Lyakhovich, V. V. (1972). *Life Sci.* 11, 1045.

Tukey, J. W. (1965). Chairman, Restoring the Quality of our Environment. Report of the Environmental Pollution Panel of the President's Science Advisory Committee, 317 pages. U.S. Government Printing Office, Washington, D.C.

Wills, E. D. (1972). *Biochem. Pharmacol.* 21, 239.

Witting, L. A. (1965). *J. Amer. Oil Chemists' Soc.* 42, 908.

The Effect of Temperature Changes on Lipids and Proteins of Biological Membranes

ROLAND C. ALOIA, AND GEORGE ROUSER

Summary

Three types of phase transitions have been observed in biological membranes. Two are related solely to lipid, and one appears to be related to conformational changes in protein. One of the lipid transitions is the well documented fluid to solid state transition observed in many bacterial cell membranes, which is measured by differential scanning calorimetry as well as other physical methods, enzyme activity measurements, and transport rates across membranes. The other type of lipid transition which we designate as a Critical Viscosity or Critical Volume Transition, arises from an increase in the interaction between lipid molecules through double bonds of unsaturated fatty acids resulting in their cooperative movement as a more viscous fluid as opposed to the transition to the solid state. This type of transition is not detectable by differential scanning calorimetry, although it is detectable by other physical methods and rate changes in enzyme and transport processes.

It is commonly assumed that the high liquid to solid transition of more saturated molecular species in membranes is lowered by cholesterol molecules packing between the phospholipid acyl chains. Evidence against this concept is reviewed. It is suggested that cholesterol and phospholipids in biological membranes occur in separate compartments and that the liquid to solid phase transition temperature of animal cell membranes is lowered by the lipids adopting the twisted conformation proposed by Vandenheuval.

The temperature at which an organism is able to grow or survive is generally associated with the absence of any kind of phase transition above this temperature. The absence of phase transitions is correlated with disorder producing factors. A reduction in temperature is associated with an increase in these factors which produce disorder in the bulk phase lipid and thus reduce the temperature at which the Critical Viscosity change or the transition to the solid state is possible. These factors include cis-double bonds, branched chain fatty acids, cyclopropane and cyclopropene fatty acids, short acyl chains and bulky molecules such as bromostearate.

I. Introduction

Many organisms are able to survive large environmental temperature reductions without suffering permanent damage or change. Many warm-blooded animals, which normally maintain a constant body temperature of about 37°C, can survive reductions in body temperature down to about 15°C before their heart stops beating (Hensel et al., 1973). In contrast, some warm-blooded animals are able to hibernate. They can reduce their body temperature to as low as 1°C for periods of up to several weeks (Pengelley, 1967) without ill effects. The nature of the changes in membrane components as a function of temperature are of great interest because they involve the ability of organisms to grow and survive under adverse circumstances. The factors involved in these important responses are considered in this report.

II. Liquid to Solid Phase Transitions

The numerous studies to date on the response of membranes to temperature changes have shown that the physical state of the lipids is generally a major factor. When the log of the activity of a soluble enzyme is plotted against the reciprocal of the absolute temperature, a straight line relationship is obtained with a gradual reduction in activity as the temperature is lowered (Lee and Gear, 1974; Raison, 1972; Lenaz et al., 1972). When the activity of a membrane-bound enzyme or transport process is plotted (Arrhenius plot), however, a break or discontinuity is generally observed which denotes a phase transition with the activation energy changing abruptly at a characteristic temperature (Raison, 1972; Lyons, 1972).

There are two different types of lipid phase transitions detectable in biological membranes. The first is the well documented fluid to solid transition detected by differential scanning calorimetry (DSC), as well as other physical methods. The second type is one which does not involve a fluid to solid phase change and is not detectable by DSC, although it is detectable by electron spin resonance probes, X-ray diffraction, enzyme assay, and other physical techniques.

Analysis of the phase transition problem is simplest in bacteria because their lipid composition is relatively simple and the types of carbon chains can be varied by growth on different media. Application of differential scanning calorimetry to bacterial membranes has disclosed, in some cases, a single transition temperature with intact cells, their isolated membranes, and the lipids extracted from these membranes (McElhaney, 1974; Reinert and Steim, 1970; Steim *et al.*, 1969), as illustrated in Fig. 1. It is clear that the transition *is related* to the change of lipid molecules from the liquid-crystalline, fluid state to a more solid or gel-like state. It is important to note, however, that the amplitude of the response with membranes is quantitatively less than that observed with lipid extracted from these membranes (Fig. 1). This indicates that interaction of lipid with protein within the membrane removes some of the lipid from the bulk phase. In general, it would appear that the bulk phase lipid unaltered by interaction with protein involves about 75 to 85% of the total phospholipid of the membrane when measured by DSC.

In lipid bilayer systems, transition temperatures can be measured by DSC and the spin label method, but spin labels may not show a transition temperature corresponding precisely to that seen by calorimetry. Some spin labels appear to perturb the region of the membrane into which they enter sufficiently to lower the transition temperature of that region. These perturbations are most pronounced at higher spin label concentrations, as is apparent with stearic acid which is found to melt at a temperature approximately 10°C higher than the transition temperature measured by a nitroxyl spin label (Melhorn *et al.*, 1973). When the appropriate spin label concentrations are used, however, the phase transitions observed in some bacterial membranes with the spin label method, as well as phase transitions determined by enzyme assay and measurement of transport processes, fall within the range of the

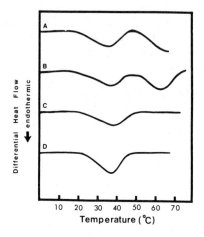

Fig. 1. (A) *Differential calorimeter scan of cells of* Mycoplasma laidlawii *in the logarithmic phase in growth medium; (B) Initial scan of membranes from the same preparation of cells shown in (A), suspended in buffer; (C) Second scan of the same membrane preparation after denaturation of protein; (D) Scan of protein-free lipid-extracted from membranes and suspended in buffer. Redrawn from data of Reinert and Steim,* Science *168, 1580 (1970).*

DSC-detectable fluid to solid state transitions. When two different phase transition temperatures are observed for bacterial membranes by enzyme assay or with spin labels at appropriate concentrations, it would appear that in some cases the higher temperature is the beginning of the transition resulting from some of the molecular species entering the solid state, and the lower temperature represents the completion of the transition to the solid state of all molecular species of phospholipid. This relationship between phase transitions detectable by enzyme assay, spin labels or measurement of transport processes and the fluid to solid, DSC-detectable transition has been demonstrated for membranes of both *Acholeplasma laidlawii* and *Escherichia coli* (McElhaney, 1974; Heast *et al.*, 1974; Dekruyff *et al.*, 1973; Shimshick *et al.*, 1973a; Steim *et al.*, 1969; Overath, 1970). Although enzymes and transport systems of bacteria are generally most active when the lipids of the membranes are in a fluid state, growth of bacterial cells is nevertheless possible with some of the membrane lipid in the solid state. Thus, in one study it was estimated that *Acholeplasma* cells could grow at the optimal rate when up to 50% of the membrane lipid was in the solid state. As the amount of solid phase was increased, the growth rate decreased steadily to zero at 90% (McElhaney, 1974).

When the liquid to solid transition temperature of a single molecular species of phospholipid is measured with a spin probe such as TEMPO (2,2,6,6-tetramethylpiperidine-1-oxyl), which is soluble in both the aqueous and hydrocarbon phases; a single transition is observed which is characteristic of the polar head group and the length and degree of unsaturation of the acyl chains (Grant *et al.*, 1974). When two different molecular species with different transition temperatures are mixed, two transition temperatures are observed with the TEMPO spin label. These are related to the transition of each molecular species, the exact values depending upon the concentration of each phospholipid (Shimshick and McConnell, 1973b). Phase diagrams can be constructed from such data (Fig. 2). Whereas dipalmitoyl phosphatidylcholine (DPPC, 16:0) has a transition temperature of 40°C and dielaidoyl phosphatidylcholine (DEPC, 18:1) has a transition at 12°C, a 3:1 molar mixture of DPPC and DEPC has transition temperature of 38° and 22°C and a 1:1 molar mixture has transition temperatures of 32° and 14°C (Grant *et al.*, 1974).

III. Freeze-Fracture Electron Microscopy and Phase Transitions

When an equimolar mixture of DPPC and DEPC was examined by freeze-fracture electron microscopy employing rapid freezing, it was observed that above the highest spin label-detectable phase transition temperature, the fracture faces appear smooth surfaced. In the region between the two transition temperatures, there are two separate fracture face appearances; one is smooth and characteristic of the fluid molecular species, while the other exhibits a banded structural pattern characteristic of the solid phase packing of the more saturated of the two species. Finally, below the second phase transition temperature all of the lipid is in the solid state, and only a banded pattern characteristic of the solid phase packing is observed (Grant *et al.*, 1974). This banded pattern is observed with

229

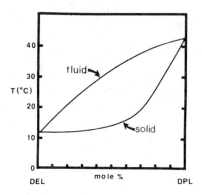

Fig. 2. Fluid/gel phase diagram for hydrated dielaidoyl/ dipalmitoyl phosphatidylcholine mixtures. The x-axis shows the mole ratio of the phospholipid mixture, ranging from pure dielaidoyl (DEL) to pure dipalmitoyl phosphatidylcholine (DPL). Conditions corresponding to points above the fluid represent totally fluid lipid mixtures, while points below the solid represent totally solid lipid. For points between these two curves, fluid and solid coexist, the domain compositions being predicted by the intersection points with the fluid and solid, respectively, of a horizontal through the point. Redrawn from data of Grant et al., Biochim. Biophys. Acta 363, 151 (1974).

phosphatidylcholine (lecithin), possibly due to a rearrangement of the polar head group in the solid state since phosphatidylethanolamine does not exhibit such banding patterns (Ververgaert *et al.*, 1973). The lipid regions of biological membranes appear to show only the smooth pattern after freeze fracture.

Freeze-fracture of membranes of both procaryotic and eucaryotic cells discloses the presence of intramembranous particles (IMPs). IMP distribution is a function of temperature (Heast *et al.*, 1974; Kleeman and McConnell, 1974; Wunderlich *et al.*, 1973; James and Branton, 1973). When *E. coli* cells are quenched sufficiently rapidly from above the phase transition temperature of their constituent lipids, a normal, seemingly "random" (no definite repeating

pattern) appearance of IMPs is seen in the fracture plane.
As the temperature is reduced and cells are quenched from
temperatures between the two lipid phase transition temperatures, increasing degrees of clumping or clustering
are observed. Finally, when cells are quenched from below
the lower phase transition, the most complete clustering
of IMPs is seen (Heast et al., 1974). IMP clustering or
clumping of this nature can be explained simply as follows.
Lipid in some regions of the membrane becomes relatively
more viscous as temperature is reduced. As the more mobile
region moves away from the more viscous region, more IMPs
may approach each other in close proximity. There appears
to be a delicate balance between the forces holding the
IMPs in normal distribution. These forces can become
unbalanced by decreasing the temperature, as mentioned
above, which thus causes IMP clustering (Heast et al.,
1974), or conversely, by raising the temperature. In
Acholeplasma cells grown on lauric acid at 25°C, the lipid
regions are sufficiently viscous to prevent extensive particle clustering. However, when the temperature is raised
to 37°C, that is, slightly above a spin label–determined
phase transition temperature, the lipid region becomes
sufficiently fluid to allow particle clustering (James and
Branton, 1973).

IV. Alteration of Phase Transitions

In bacterial systems, when the fatty acids available in
the medium are sufficiently unsaturated, the transition
temperature of the bulk phase lipid determined by calorimetry, can be lowered to well below 0°C (McElhaney, 1974).
However, despite this low transition, growth of Acholeplasma ceases at approximately 8°C (McElhaney, 1974). This
indicates that the minimal temperature of growth in this
organism is a characteristic of the general organization
of the membrane.

In bacterial and yeast membrane systems, it is amply
documented that growth at reduced temperatures changes the
types of acyl chains of lipids. Growth at lower temperatures can be associated with an increase in the amount of
branched chains, the introduction of cyclopropane or cyclopropene rings, shortening of carbon chain lengths, or increased unsaturation. All of these changes lower the temperature at which the lipid solidifies (Sousa et al.,
1974; McElhaney et al., 1973; Thorpe and Ratledge, 1973;

Kates and Paradis, 1973; Heast *et al.*, 1972; Okuyama, 1969), by increasing disorder in the bulk phase lipid association. That this is the case is indicated by the observation that bromostearate can satisfy the unsaturated fatty acid requirements of an *E. coli* mutant (Fox and Tsukagoshi, 1972). Similarly, incorporation of the hydrophobic, bulky molecule, adamantane into yeast membrane lipids lowers the transition temperature for physiological processes and alters spin label mobility (Eletr *et al.*, 1974).

The liquid to solid phase transition characteristic of a particular molecular species of phospholipid can be altered by addition of cholesterol to a lipid bilayer system *in vitro*. As the cholesterol content is increased, the intensity of the DSC response and the sharpness of the break on an Arrhenius plot are decreased and are no longer apparent at 32 moles % or above (Oldfield and Chapman, 1972; Ladbrooke and Chapman, 1969). This has been clearly shown (Fig. 3) in model lipid systems such as 1,2 dipalmitoyl-L-lecithin-cholesterol mixtures, in which the peak height is reduced and the peak base width is increased with increasing cholesterol content (Ladbrooke *et al.*, 1968a). Thus, cholesterol lowers the fluid to solid transition temperature of the bilayer system.

The transition temperature of enzyme activities of biological membranes of microorganisms that do not normally contain sterol can also be reduced by the inclusion of cholesterol. When cholesterol was incorporated to a level of 9 moles % into the membranes of *Acholeplasma laidlawii* grown on cholesterol and elaidic acid, the temperature of the Arrhenius discontinuity for ATPase activity was found to be 6°C lower than that from cells grown on elaidate alone (Dekruyff *et al.*, 1973). Similarly, in yeast mitochondria, the temperature of the Arrhenius breaks of ATPase activity was found to decrease from 34 to 26°C when the content of ergosterol increased from less than 1% to about 5%, and a further reduction from 26° to 18°C was observed when the sterol content was increased to about 10% (Cobon and Haslam, 1973).

V. Critical Viscosity or Critical Volume Transition

Although the liquid to solid phase transitions (measured by DSC) are observed in animal cell membranes only

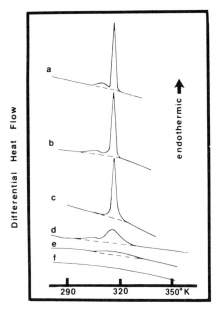

Fig. 3. *DSC curves of 50 weight % dispersions in water of 1,2-dipalmitoyl-L-lecithin-cholesterol mixtures containing (a) 0.0 mole %, (b) 5.0 mole %, (c) 12.5 mole %, (d) 20.0 mole %, (e) 32 mole %, and (f) 50.0 mole % cholesterol. Redrawn from data of Ladbrooke and Chapman, Lipids 3, 304 (1969).*

near or below 0°C (Blazyk and Steim, 1972), Arrhenius plots of enzyme activity, spin probe mobility, and transport processes of many animal cell membranes exhibit discontinuities well above 0°C that are not liquid to solid transitions. We term these Critical Viscosity (Critical Volume) transitions. Spin labels and enzyme activity measurements of mitochondria and microsomes disclose breaks in Arrhenius plots 20° to 30°C above the calorimetrically-determined fluid-solid state transitions for these membranes (Raison and McMurchie, 1974; McMurchie *et al.*, 1973; Raison, 1972; Lyons, 1972). As is seen in Fig. 4A, one break in the Arrhenius plot is easily observed and a second break is suggested. However, numerous data points are required to prove the discontinuity as shown in Fig. 4B in which the lines in Fig. 4A are redrawn. It is thus not surprising that some earlier reports on the same membrane system indicated only one discontinuity (see Shimshick and Mc-Connell, 1973b; Linden *et al.*, 1973; Fox and Tsukagoshi, 1972; Raison and Lyons, 1971; Lyons and Raison, 1970).

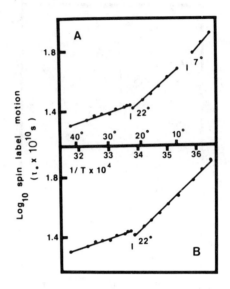

Fig. 4. Arrhenius plots of the motion of the spin label M12NS infused into rat liver endoplasmic reticulum membranes. The calculated values for the Arrhenius activation energy of motion in each temperature range from 45°C are 21.1, 30, and 41 kc/mole. Redrawn from data of Raison and McMurchie, Biochim. Biophys. Acta 363, 135 (1974).

Phase transitions well above 0°C were also observed with membranes of bacteria grown on unsaturated fatty acids that reduce the liquid to solid transition to well below 0°C. For example, *Acholeplasma* cells with a membrane lipid composition of approximately 60 to 66% oleic acid (McElhaney, 1974; Tourtellotte *et al.*, 1970), have a liquid to solid state transition around -15 to -20°C, when measured by DSC or X-ray diffraction (Engleman, 1971; Steim *et al.*, 1969), yet spin labels undergo a transition at about 20°C (Rottem *et al.*, 1970). Similarly, with *E. coli* containing 50 to 58% oleic acid in their membranes by growth on oleic acid medium (Overath and Trauble, 1973; Heast *et al.*, 1972; Overath *et al.*, 1970), no DSC-detectable phase transition could be observed above 0°C, although a transition for dichloroindolphenol reductase was seen at 18°C (Heast *et al.*, 1974). Also with yeast cell membranes containing 78% oleic acid, changes in spin label mobility indicate a transition at about 16°C (Eletr and Keith, 1972) and yeast cells containing between 56 to 72% linolenic acid in their membranes show spin label detectable transitions at approximately 10°C (James *et al.*, 1972). These transitions are well above the fluid to solid state transition.

Phase transitions above the fluid-solid state transition have also been observed in model systems and animal cell membranes. When the spin label TEMPO was added to an aqueous dispersion of dioleyl phosphatidylcholine (DOPC), a discontinuity at 30°C was found (Lee *et al.*, 1974). Additionally, purified rabbit muscle Ca^{++}-dependent ATPase with its native lipid, or when reconstituted with DOPC replacing the natural lipid, shows a break in an Arrhenius plot of enzyme activity at 29°C (Lee *et al.*, 1974). Differential scanning calorimetry shows a fluid-solid state transition for DOPC centered around -22°C, and thus phase transitions at approximately 30°C must result from some other phenomenon.

Since transitions above the liquid to solid transition are observed only with molecular species containing unsaturated fatty acids, increased interaction of carbon chains through double bonds causing molecules to move together with a decrease in volume and an increase in viscosity, is the most obvious reason for the phase transition. Since motion is not stopped, as in the liquid to solid phase transition, this type of transition is not detectable by DSC, although it is detectable by other physical methods, as well as by enzyme activity and transport rate measurements. It is a characteristic of membranes and model systems containing unsaturated fatty acids and is thus seen, as cited above, in bacterial membranes when saturated fatty acids are replaced by unsaturated species.

When unsaturated fatty acids occur in both the 1 and 2 positions, each phospholipid molecule can interact with all of its neighbors through double bonds. Although this type of molecular species does occur in many membranes, it does not appear in significant amount in others such as the Ca^{++} pump of sarcoplasmic reticulum (Marai and Kuksis, 1973) that show the Critical Viscosity type of phase transition. It thus appears that molecular species containing one polyunsaturated fatty acid and one saturated fatty acid show the phenomenon. When molecules on opposite sides of the bilayer interdigitate, all molecules are effectively linked together when double bonds occur only in the fatty acids at the 2-position. Interdigitation appears to be a very general phenomenon caused by a difference in the

length of the two acyl chains. It is most obvious for
sphingolipids, particularly with molecules that contain
sphingosine and 24 carbon fatty acids, since in such
species, sphingosine is equivalent to a 14 carbon fatty
acid in a glycerophospholipid. It appears that the acyl
chains of most molecular species of glycerophospholipids
are different in length since 16 and 18 carbon fatty acids
frequently appear in the same molecules with 20 and 22
carbon acids (Kuksis et al., 1968). In addition, molecular
species containing the same fatty acids in both positions
may not give molecules with the same chain lengths since
X-ray diffraction has disclosed a mismatch of about three
carbon atoms in the solid state (Hitchcock et al., 1974).

VI. Role of Cholesterol in Lipid Phase Transitions
of Animal Cell Membranes

It is commonly assumed that cholesterol molecules pack
between those of phospholipids and lower the liquid to
solid phase transition temperature of those molecular
species that in vitro, in the absence of cholesterol, show
higher transition temperatures than those of biological
membranes. However, a number of observations are difficult
to reconcile with this concept. Thus, it is difficult to
see why different membranes from the same type of cell
should have such grossly different cholesterol/phospholipid
molar ratios (from < 0.1 to about 0.9) except by assuming
that cholesterol and phospholipid occur in separate positions in membranes, and that the units containing choles-
terol-only, vary in amount. Lipid exchange data for human
and dog red blood cells show that cholesterol and part of
the phosphatidylcholine and sphingomyelin undergo exchange
with plasma (Reed, 1968; Murphy, 1965). Since about 40%
of the cholesterol can be removed from the membrane without a change in phospholipid composition, it appears that
cholesterol and the exchangeable phospholipids do not oc-
cupy the same space. If they did, removal of cholesterol
would be expected to increase the amount of phospholipid.
It is also difficult to see why red cell cholesterol can
undergo complete exchange, whereas phospholipids of some
species do not exchange at all (Winterbourn and Batt,
1968) or only partially (Reed, 1968), other than by their
occurrence in separate units. Also, polar lipids can re-
place each other, but cholesterol does not appear to be
involved (Rouser and Kritchevsky, 1972). Finally, it has
been observed that phospholipid molecules containing

unsaturated fatty acids in the 1 and 2-position can be cross-linked through their double bonds by reaction with osmium (Korn, 1966), and that such cross-linking destroys the fracture plane (Nermut and Ward, 1974; James and Branton, 1971).

Molecules, such as dipalmitoyl phosphatidylcholine, with a liquid to solid transition at 41°C (Phillips et al., 1969) occur in large amounts in some animal cell membranes (Montfoort et al., 1971). If cholesterol does not pack between phospholipid molecules to lower the liquid to solid transition temperature, an alternative explanation must be sought. Adoption of the twisted conformation described by Vandenheuval (1968; 1971) appears to be a reasonable alternative that should make transition to the extended solid state more difficult and thus lower the transition temperature. If this is the case for animal cell membranes, then it would appear that phospholipids in bacterial cell membranes do not pack in this twisted conformation since they can show liquid to solid transition temperatures characteristic of the lipid extracted from their membranes (Steim, 1972; Reinert and Steim, 1970; Steim et al., 1969).

VII. Protein Conformational Changes

Besides fluid to solid transitions detectable by DSC and transitions which we are denoting as Critical Viscosity or Volume transitions, it appears that breaks in Arrhenius plots can also be produced by a protein conformational change which can be transmitted to the bulk phase lipid. This is apparently the case for rabbit skeletal muscle Ca^{++}-Mg^{++}-ATPase and guinea pig liver microsomal UDP-glucuronyl transferase. Two breaks in Arrhenius plots could be detected for Ca^{++}-transport and steady state Ca^{++}-dependent ATPase activity (Inesi et al., 1973). The role of protein was disclosed as follows: lipophilic spin probes were able to detect both breaks in Arrhenius plots, except after heat treatment to denature protein, when the upper break was no longer observed. That this upper break was due to protein was confirmed by the use of protein-bound, as well as sulfhydryl-sensitive spin labels which could only detect the Arrhenius break at the upper temperature (Inesi et al., 1973; Eletr and Inesi, 1972). UDP-glucuronyl transferase activity also shows two breaks on an Arrhenius plot (Eletr et al., 1973). The lower break in enzyme activity can be eliminated by phospholipase A and, therefore, appears to be due to a lipid phase transition. The upper break could be eliminated by heat treatment and, therefore, appears to be due to protein. The protein conformational change is apparently translated to the lipid phase since both Arrhenius breaks are seen when the spin label probe 6N11 is used (Eletr *et al.*, 1973).

VIII. Cold Adaptation and Hibernation

As can be expected, membranes from plant and animal species capable of growth or survival at lower temperatures, fail to exhibit breaks in Arrhenius plots of lipid-associated enzyme activity and spin label mobility. This has been demonstrated in numerous plant tissues, such as beet roots, potato tubers, peas, and cauliflower (Raison, 1972; Lyons, 1972), and for toad and fish mitochondrial membranes (McMurchie *et al.*, 1973; Raison and Lyons, 1971; Lyons and Raison, 1970; Richardson and Tappel, 1963). Also no Arrhenius plot discontinuities were detected with enzyme activity measurements or spin labels in toad heart mitochondria from approximately 5 to 35°C (McMurchie *et al.*, 1973).

The absence of phase transitions in these plant and animal tissues has been correlated with the degree of fatty acyl unsaturation (Hazel and Prosser, 1974; Lyons, 1973; De La Roche *et al.*, 1973). In gill mitochondria from 10°C-adapted goldfish, there are distinct changes in phospholipid class composition which are accompanied by an increase in polyunsaturated and a decrease in saturated fatty acids (Caldwell and Vernberg, 1970). Similarly, fatty acids with 4, 5, and 6 double bonds increased in goldfish brain after adaptation to lower temperatures (Roots, 1968). The increase in unsaturation is apparently of such a nature as to disrupt the hydrocarbon double bond interaction of membrane phospholipids and thereby abolish the Critical Viscosity Transition normally observed with decreasing temperatures. It appears that the double bonds in adjacent molecules are not positioned properly for interaction. As might be anticipated, changes in the reverse direction, i.e., a decrease in unsaturation, were found in red blood cells of hamsters exposed continuously to the abnormally high environmental temperature of 35°C (Kuiper *et al.*, 1971).

Mammals capable of hibernation have the capacity to survive at reduced body temperatures of about $1^{\circ}C$ for intervals of 2 to 4 weeks and experience no apparent harmful effects (Pengelley, 1967). The heart beat of the hibernating ground squirrel decreases from about 350 beats per minute at $37^{\circ}C$ to about 2 beats per minute at $1^{\circ}C$ (Johansson, 1967). In sharp contrast to this capacity to function at low temperatures, the hearts of mammals incapable of hibernation undergo ventricular fibrillation and stop beating at about $15^{\circ}C$ (Hensel, 1973). These observations are in line with what has been discussed above for lipid phase transitions. Breaks at $20^{\circ}C$ have been observed in Arrhenius plots of rabbit heart beat, succinate oxidase activity and spin label mobility. Similar transitions at $20^{\circ}C$ were also found for $Na^{+}-K^{+}$ ATPase activity and spin label mobility of a combined endoplasmic reticulum-plasma membrane preparation from the rabbit heart (Raison and McMurchie, 1974).

In mammals capable of, but unprepared for hibernation (body temperature of $37^{\circ}C$), mitochondrial succinate oxidase shows an Arrhenius plot-break at 22° or $23^{\circ}C$ as seen with animals incapable of hibernation. On the other hand, the heart of mammals prepared for hibernation continues to beat as temperature is reduced and a linear Arrhenius plot for succinate oxidase is observed (Lyons, 1972).

Analysis of changes in phospholipids of hibernating ground squirrel hearts showed an increase (3.5-fold) of lysophospholipids (Aloia et al., 1974). This is shown in histogram form in Fig. 5 in which the bars on the right represent the phospholipids of the hibernating squirrel and those on the left the phospholipids of the active squirrel capable of, but unprepared for, hibernation (Aloia et al., 1974).

Keith et al. (1975) have analyzed the effect of lyso-glycerophosphatides on the physical state of the membrane lipids as a function of temperature. Arrhenius plots were made of the rotational correlation times for the spin labels 2N12 and 2N8 added to liver mitochondria and the phospholipids from whole heart and from heart and liver mitochondria from active and from hibernating ground squirrels. As expected, a straight line Arrhenius plot was obtained from the hibernating squirrel tissues. Similarly, as expected, the Arrhenius plot from the active ground squirrel showed a discontinuity at temperatures between

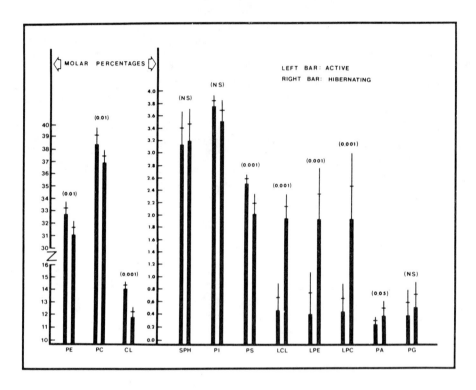

Fig. 5. Histogram illustrating the molar percentage values of phospholipid classes of active and hibernating ground squirrel hearts. The mean value (cross hatch), standard deviation (thin vertical line), and level of significance (parentheses) are indicated. Probability was determined by nonpaired T-test comparing active with hibernating animals (NS = not significant). Abbreviations: PE = phosphatidylethanolamine; PC = phosphatidylcholine; DPG = diphosphatidyl glycerol; SPH = sphingomyelin; PI = phosphatidylinositol; PS = phosphatidylserine; LDPG = lysodiphosphatidyl glycerol; LPE = lysophosphatidyl ethanolamine; LPC = lysophosphatidyl choline; PA = phosphatidic acid; PG = phosphatidyl glycerol.

21° and 23°C for mitochondria and extracted lipids, with an increase in activation energy below the transition temperature (Fig. 6). However, by adding 7 moles % egg yolk lysolecithin (only saturated fatty acids) to the phospholipids from the active ground squirrel (to make the total content

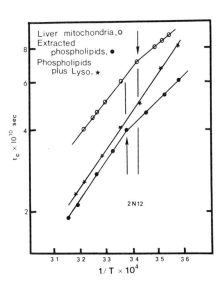

Fig. 6. Mitochondria and extracted phospholipids from active squirrel liver. All samples were spin labeled with 2N12 immediately before analysis. o, liver mitochondria; •, phospholipids extracted from liver mitochondria; ★, same extracted liver mitochondrial phospholipids with 7 mole % of lysolecithin added.

of lysophosphatides equal to that found during hibernation), the discontinuity was eliminated and a linear plot was produced (Keith *et al.*, 1975). This is direct physical evidence that physiological concentrations of lysoglycero-phosphatides alter the disorder properties of membrane lipids. The presence of lysoglycerophosphatides is expected to decrease the hydrocarbon density sufficiently to allow for greater thermal molecular motion at reduced temperatures and decrease interaction through double bonds.

Recent studies of Na^+-K^+-ATPase also indicate the importance of lysoglycerophosphatides. The Arrhenius breaks in ATPase enzyme activity at 18 and 20°C of rabbit renal cortical microsomes and ox brain microsomes, were eliminated by brief treatment with phospholipase A_2 (Charnock et al., 1973; Taniguchi and Iito, 1972, respectively). Since the reaction medium contained bovine serum albumin, which binds free fatty acids more avidly than lysophospholipids (Fleischer and Fleischer, 1967), and the enzyme preparations were not further washed with albumin-containing buffers that would remove lysophospholipids, it would appear that the effect of abolishing the phase transition is due to the presence of lysoglycerophosphatides.

ACKNOWLEDGMENTS

We would like to gratefully acknowledge the generous assistance from the National Institutes of Health Grant Number HL 13532-04, and intramural grants from the University of California at Riverside to Dr. E. T. Pengelley, research funds from the American Heart Association, Riverside, California affiliate to Dr. R. C. Aloia and grants NS 01847 and 06237 from the National Institute of Neurological Diseases and Stroke to Dr. G. Rouser.

References

Aloia, R. C., Pengelley, E. T., Bolen, J., and Rouser, G. (1974). *Lipids* 9, 993.

Blazyk, J. F., and Steim, J. M. (1972). *Biochim. Biophys. Acta* 266, 737.

Caldwell, R. S., and Vernberg, F. J. (1970). *Comp. Biochem. Physiol.* 34, 179.

Charnock, J. S., Cook, D. A., Almeida, A. F., and To, R. (1973). *Arch. Biochem. Biophys.* 159, 393.

Cobon, G. S., and Haslam, J. M. (1973). *Biochem. Biophys. Res. Commun.* 52, 320.

Dekruyff, B., Van Dijck, P. W. M., Goldbach, R. W., Demel, R. A., and Van Deenen, L. L. M. (1973). *Biochim. Biophys. Acta* 330, 269.

De La Roche, I. A., Andrews, C. J., and Kates, M. (1973). *Plant Physiol.* 51, 468.

Eletr, S., and Inesi, G. (1972). *Biochim. Biophys. Acta* 290, 178.

Eletr, S., and Keith, A. D. (1972). *P.N.A.S.* 69, 1353.
Eletr, S., Williams, M. A., Watkins, T., and Keith, A. D. (1974). *Biochim. Biophys. Acta* 339, 190.
Eletr, S., Zakim, D., and Vessey, D. A. (1973). *J. Mol. Biol.* 78, 351.
Engleman, D. M. (1971). *J. Mol. Biol.* 58, 153.
Fleischer, S., and Fleischer, B. (1967). *In* "Methods in Enzymology" (R. W. Estabrook and M. E. Pullman, eds.), p. 406, v. 10. Academic Press, New York.
Fox, C. F., and Tsukagoshi, N. (1972). *In* "Membrane Research" (C. F. Fox, ed.), p. 145. Academic Press, New York.
Gottlieb, M. H., and Eanes, E. D. (1974). *Biochim. Biophys. Acta* 373, 519.
Grant, C. W. M., Wu, S. H. W., and Connell, H. M. (1974). *Biochim. Biophys. Acta* 363, 151.
Hazel, J. R., and Prosser, L. (1974). *Physiol. Rev.*, July.
Heast, C. W. M., DeGier, J., VanEs, G. A., Verkleij, J., and Van Deenen, L. L. M. (1972). *Biochim. Biophys. Acta* 288, 43.
Heast, C. W. M., Verkleiu, A. J., DeGier, J., Scheik, R., Ververgaert, P. H. J., and Van Deenen, L. L. M. (1974). *Biochim. Biophys. Acta* 356, 17.
Hensel, H., Bruck, K., and Raths, P. (1973). *In* "Temperature and Life" (H. Precht, J. Christophersen, H. Hensel and W. Larcher, eds.), p. 505. Springer-Verlag, Berlin.
Hitchcock, P. B., Mason, R., Thomas, K. M., and Shipley, G. G. (1974). *P.N.A.S.* 71, 3036.
Inesi, G., Millman, M., and Eletr, S. (1973). *J. Mol. Biol.* 81, 483.
James, R., and Branton, D. (1971). *Biochim. Biophys. Acta* 233, 504.
James, R., and Branton, D. (1973). *Biochim. Biophys. Acta* 323, 378.
James, R., Branton, D., Wisnieski, B., and Keith, A. (1972). *J. Supremol. Str.* 1, 38.
Johansson, B. W. (1967). *In* "Mammalian Hibernation III" (K. C. Fisher *et al.*, eds.), p. 200. Oliver and Boyd, London.
Kates, M., and Paradis, M. (1973). *Can. J. Biochem.* 51, 184.
Keith, A. D., Aloia, R. C., Lyons, J., Snipes, W., Pengelley, E. T. (1975). *Biochim. Biophys. Acta* 394, 204.
Kleeman, W., and McConnell, H. M. (1974). *Biochim. Biophys. Acta* 345, 220.

Korn, E. D. (1966). *Biochim. Biophys. Acta* 116, 235.

Kuiper, P. J. C., Livne, A., and Meyerstein, N. (1971). *Biochim. Biophys. Acta* 248, 300.

Kuksis, A., Marai, L., Breckenridge, W. C., Gornall, D. A., and Stachnyk, O. (1968). *Can. J. Physiol. Pharmacol.* 46, 511.

Ladbrooke, B. D., and Chapman, D. (1969). *Chem. Phys. Lipids* 3, 304.

Ladbrooke, B. D., Williams, R. M., and Chapman, D. (1968a). *Biochim. Biophys. Acta* 150, 333.

Ladbrooke, B. D., Jenkinson, T. J., Kamat, V. B., and Chapman, D. (1968b). *Biochim. Biophys. Acta* 164, 101.

Lee, A. G., Birdsall, N. J. M., Metcalfe, J. C., Toon, P. A., and Warren, G. B. (1974). *Biochem.* 13, 3699.

Lee, M. P., and Gear, A. R. L. (1974). *J. Biol. Chem.* 249, 7541.

Lenaz, G., Sechi, A. M., Parenti-Castelli, G., Landi, L., and Bertoli, E. (1972). *Biochem. Biophys. Res. Commun.* 49, 536.

Linden, C. D., Wright, K. L., McConnell, H. M., and Fox, C. F. (1973). *P.N.A.S.* 70, 2271.

Lyons, J. M. (1972). *Cryobiol.* 9, 341.

Lyons, J. M. (1973). *Ann. Rev. Plant Physiol.* 24, 445.

Lyons, J. M., and Raison, J. K. (1970). *Comp. Biochem. Physiol.* 37, 405.

Marai, L., and Kuksis, A. (1973). *Can. J. Biochem.* 51, 1365.

McElhaney, R. N. (1974). *J. Mol. Biol.* 84, 145.

McElhaney, R. N., DeGier, J., and Van Den Neut-Kok, E. C. M. (1973). *Biochim. Biophys. Acta* 298, 500.

McMurchie, E. J., Raison, J. K., and Cairncross, K. D. (1973). *Comp. Biochem. Physiol.* 44B, 1017.

Melhorn, R., Snipes, W., and Keith, A. (1973). *Biophys. J.* 13, 1223.

Montfoort, A., Van Golde, L. M. G., and Van Deenen, L. L. M. (1971). *Biochim. Biophys. Acta* 231, 335.

Murphy, J. R. (1965). *J. Lab. Clin. Med.* 65, 756.

Nermut, M. V., and Ward, B. J. (1974). *J. Microsc.* 102, 29.

Okuyama, H. (1969). *Biochim. Biophys. Acta* 176, 125.

Oldfield, E., and Chapman, D. (1972). *FEBS Letters* 23, 285.

Overath, P., and Trauble, H. (1973). *Biochem.* 12, 2625.

Overath, P., Schairer, H. U., and Stoffel, W. (1970). *P.N.A.S.* 67, 606.

Pengelley, E. T. (1967). *In* "Mammalian Hibernation III" (K. C. Fisher *et al.*, eds.), p. l. Oliver and Boyd, London.

Phillips, M. C., Williams, R. M., and Chapman, D. (1969). *Chem. Phys. Lipids* 3, 234.

Raison, J. K. (1972). *Bioenergetics* 4, 559.

Raison, J. K., and Lyons, J. M. (1971). *P.N.A.S.* 68, 2092.

Raison, J. K., and McMurchie, E. J. (1974). *Biochim. Biophys. Acta* 363, 135.

Rand, R. P., and Pangborn. (1973). *Biochim. Biophys. Acta* 318, 299.

Reed, C. F. (1968). *J. Clin. Invest.* 47, 749.

Reinert, J. C., and Steim, J. M. (1970). *Science* 168, 1580.

Richardson, T., and Tappel, A. L. (1963). *J. Cell Biol.* 13, 43.

Roots, B. I. (1968). *Comp. Biochem. Physiol.* 25, 457.

Rottem, S., Hubbell, W. L., Hayflick, L., and McConnell, H. M. (1970). *Biochim. Biophys. Acta* 219, 104.

Rouser, G., and Kritchevsky, G. (1972). *In* "Sphingolipids, Sphingolipidoses, and Allied Disorders" (B. W. Volk and S. M. Aronson, eds.), p. 101. Plenum Press, New York.

Shimshick, E. J., Kleeman, W., Hubbell, W. L., and McConnell, H. M. (1973a). *J. Supramol. Str.* 1, 285.

Shimshick, E. J., and McConnell, H. M. (1973b). *Biochem. Biophys. Res. Commun.* 53, 446.

Sousa, K. A., Kostin, L. L., and Tyson, B. J. (1974). *Arch. Microbiol.* 97, 89.

Steim, J. M. (1972). *Fed. Eup. Biochem. Soc. Proc.* 28, 185.

Steim, J. M., Tourtellotte, M. E., Reinert, J. C., McElhaney, R. N., and Rader, R. L. (1969). *P.N.A.S.* 63, 104.

Taniguchi, K., and Iito, S. (1972). *Biochim. Biophys. Acta* 274, 536.

Thorpe, R. F., and Ratledge, C. (1973). *J. Gen. Micro.* 78, 203.

Tourtellotte, M. E., Branton, D., and Keith, A. (1970). *P.N.A.S.* 66, 909.

Vandenheuval, F. A. (1968). *Chem. Phys. Lipids* 2, 372.

Vandenheuval, F. A. (1971). *In* "Advances in Lipid Research" (R. Paoletti and D. Kritchevsky, eds.), p. 161. Academic Press, New York.

Ververgaert, P. H. J. Th., Verkeij, A. J., Elbers, P. F., and Van Deenen, L. L. M. (1973). *Biochim. Biophys. Acta* 311, 320.

Winterbourn, C. C., and Batt, R. D. (1968). *Biochim. Biophys. Acta* 152, 412.

Wunderlich, F., Speth, V., Batz, W., and Kleinig, K. (1973). *Biochim. Biophys. Acta* 298, 39.

A 5
B 6
C 7
D 8
E 9
F 0
G 1
H 2
I 3
J 4